A Clinicians Guide to Clinical Research

A Clinicians Guide to Clinical Research

John Somberg, MD

American Institute Publishing

Division of American Institute Therapeutics
21 N Skokie Hwy, Suite G3
Lake Bluff, IL 60044

ISBN: 978-1-7368527-1-2

Library of Congress Control Number: 2022944654

Printed in the US by Amazon Kindle Direct Publishing

Dedication

To the clinical medical investigators whose tireless work strives to alleviate suffering and prolong life.

John Somberg MD
Biographical Sketch

Dr. John Somberg was born in NYC, graduated New York University with a BA in 1970, New York Medical College in 1974 with an MD degree and completed his Cardiology Fellowship at Harvard Medical School, Peter Bent Brigham Hospital in 1978. He served as an instructor Department of Medicine Harvard Medical School, Director of the Clinical Cardiac Arrhythmia Service at Albert Einstein College of Medicine in NY, was the Chief of Cardiology Chicago Medical School and was the Chief Division of Clinical Pharmacology, Professor of Cardiology, Medicine and Pharmacology at Rush University in Chicago, IL till his retirement as Emeritus Professor in June 2019. Dr. Somberg was also the Director of the Masters Program in Clinical Research at Rush University. Dr. Somberg is a career clinical investigator, serving as a PI in over 100 Phase I, Phase II and Phase III clinical trials. He founded and organized a course with the Cardio Renal Division of the FDA for over 25 years and has been a basic and clinical investigator in the area of anti-arrhythmic pharmacology for the past 35 years. Currently, Dr. Somberg is an advisor on the Circulatory Device FDA Advisory Committee. Dr. Somberg's involvement in drug development and as an advisor to FDA has lead him to teach at Rush University, a course on Drug & Device Development, the U.S. Regulatory Process, as part of the Masters in Clinical Research Program. He also taught Clinical Trial Design I and Clinical Trials II. Dr. Somberg has published 250 peer reviewed publications. He was the Editor of the Journal of Clinical Pharmacology for 10 years, then founder and was the Editor of the American Journal of Therapeutics for 20 years, published by Lippincott, Wilkins & Williams, as well as section editor of Therapeutics for the Journal Cardiology and is an editorial board member of the American J Cardiology. He is currently the Editor of Cardiology Research and has recently published a book "On the QT", a definitive text on cardiac repolarization and anti-arrhythmic therapy.

Preface

For the past 21 years I was the Program Director of the Master's in Clinical Research at Rush University. Along with the Chairman of Pharmacology – Paul Carvey, PhD, we founded the Masters in Clinical Research primarily aimed to familiarize young physicians (residents, fellows and junior attendings) with the tools necessary to undertake clinical research. The program was very successful over the years training 132 physicians who published over 800 papers. For those who stayed on at Rush these students brought in $16.5 million in grant funding to the University.

What knowledge I have of clinical research has come to me primarily through my experience as an academic clinician over my basic and clinical research career, "studying up" on problems as they arose. When I started the Master's Program at Rush University, I thought it appropriate that the future young researchers should not learn from the school of "hard lessons" as one progresses, but to have a more systematic basis of knowledge required to undertake clinical research. In the years of the program, I taught Clinical Trials I & II, Meta Analysis, Drug & Device Development: the U.S. Regulatory Process and a course on Readings in Clinical Research. For the courses on Clinical Trials I asked the students to read along with the lectures, the book by Friedman, Furberg and DeMets: Fundamentals of Clinical Trials. This book is a very good introduction to clinical research and from its 1st edition to the current 5th edition has been a very useful student resource. However, the authors present a narrow outlook on what constitutes clinical research. To them a randomized, controlled clinical trial is clinical research. Of course this leaves out the major area of observational clinical trials and the contributions those types of trials have made to medicine. While I have great respect for these authors, I strongly disagree with the narrow interpretation of what constitutes clinical research. In the course at Rush I was always able to supplement the book "Fundamentals of Clinical Trials" with other texts on epidemiology, meta-analysis, and articles with alternative viewpoints. I would also open for discussion many of their categorical positions such as one should only employ intent to that analysis as opposed to on treatment analysis, a position held by the majority of trialists today, but a position many clinicians do not subscribe. The viewpoint of those treating patients is that intention to treat analysis may lead to incorrect clinical recommendations due to incorrect research assessments since the treatment group is contaminated by non-compliers and/or dropouts. An example is the use of amiodarone in the treatment of arrhythmias in patients with heart failure where the conclusion was that therapy had no benefit. However in those who continued to take the drug benefit was observed.

This brings up two important points I must share with the reader. The first is that I have so often used Fundamentals of Clinical Trials as the starting point for my student lectures it is ingrained in my thoughts as a clinical researcher as are the disagreements with many of the statements made by these authors. Thus, if this book often echoes the contribution of Freedman, Furberg and DeMets, it attests to their contributions and in no way is meant to supplant their scholarships and diminish their contributions. This book is intended to give physicians interested in clinical research and conducting clinical trials a broad introduction with less dogma, that is more inclusive of the different types of clinical research approaches some of which are more feasible for most physicians to undertake. Very few clinical researchers in a career take part in large, randomized trials and even the ones that do, for the most part take part occasionally. Clinicians are much more likely to be involved in small studies, Phase II & Phase III clinical drug research trials or, as a validator in a device study. Physicians often will undertake a meta-analysis even if they plan to be part of a large multi-center investigation. They do this to survey the field and obtain a summary of the results of studies. Knowledge of all these areas is essential for a clinical investigator. Undertaking a meta-analysis is also a way for a young physician looking to advance a clinical academic career.

The second point I need to make clear to the reader is that I have spent my long career in academic medicine as a cardiovascular pharmacologist, cardiologist, basic and clinical electrophysiologist and have become involved in the areas of drug and device development. For this reason, most of the examples of clinical research I provide are in the area of cardiovascular medicine. I apologize for this narrow frame of reference, though I must point out that the field of cardiology has often lead in clinical research and enhanced clinical practice based on randomized controlled clinical trials. Cardiovascular medicine has been ahead of most other fields. Many of the early, seminal clinical trial methodologies needs to be taught in the context of cardiovascular research. Still there are many other areas with excellent studies and equally vexing problems that I am just not familiar with and thus can't allude to in this book.

I do hope the book covering clinical trial design, and an introduction to pharmaceutical and device research will open new areas of interest to physicians, and those looking to advance their career in academic medicine.

John Somberg MD

July 2022

Table of Contents

Chapter 1. Introduction

The practice of medicine is a most gratifying profession. Palliating or curing disease, relieving pain and suffering is what we do as physicians and is the reason many go into the field of medicine. But there is another dimension of medicine that is equally important. Evaluating what we do in a systematic way though well thought out clinical research. Evaluating new approaches to treatment, new therapies or new medical devices is a critical aspect of medicine. Without clinical research medical decisions would be based upon opinion and new approaches not properly introduced into practice. We would not have a basis for the practice of evidence-based medicine.

A physician must be well versed in current medical knowledge, but he must be able to evaluate the current and future practice guidelines for current and future therapy. Without clinical research we would be unable to determine successful approaches, those approaches of little value or those that cause harm. There are instances when the introduction of a new therapy such as penicillin for the treatment of pneumococcal pneumonia is an obvious success (though even here a small but well-designed trial was needed to show efficacy and treatment appropriate parameters). But even very good therapies as ACE inhibitors in heart failure are not obviously effective but need a controlled clinical trial to demonstrate efficacy and safety.

If one goes back in the literature in most fields in medicine one finds an evolution of how therapies and practices have been introduced. In the last few decades we see controlled clinical trials and more recently the use of meta-analysis to present an overview. The clinical trials are often adequately powered, randomized and blinded, at times with 1,000, 10,000, or even 100,000 patients. Going back to the 1970's one finds much smaller trials, often unblended, not randomized and in some fields case studies without control or standard therapy comparators. Going back even further one sees predominately case series, opinion papers by experts, and the occasional study of an agent compared to historical controls. Thus, just in the last half century the way medicine is practiced, how new therapies are introduced, and how the evidence medical practice is based upon has changed dramatically. This is all to the good making our current practice of medicine better and safer and offering much better results for our patients.

The patient benefits are also paralleled by benefits to those involved in undertaking clinical research.

"The successful translation of a basic or clinical observation into a new treatment of disease is rare in an investigator's life, but when it occurs, the personal thrill is exhilarating and the impact on society is substantial". *

Personal satisfaction is important, especially in the age of "physician burn out". Clinical research offers an outlet for the physician's interest, inquisitiveness and creativity.

---

*John Gallin: A Historical Perspective on Clinical Research; Galin, John and Ognibene, Frederick: Principles and Practice of Clinical Research, Second Edition, Academic Press, 2007.

Clinical research participants also offer career opportunities in academic medicine, the clinical research organization establishment, and employment at the National Institute of Health as well as (private grant funding organizations) or employment at the Food and Drug Administration (FDA). Knowledge of the workings of clinical research opens a number of potential career opportunities or a supplemental path combined with clinical practice.

Before we proceed to discuss the areas of knowledge that are fundamental to clinical research, some knowledge of the history of clinical investigation is appropriate.

The History of Clinical Research

There are many influences on clinical research from prior medical history. Mention is made of therapeutic intervention in what has been "handed down" from all the major civilizations. Ancient Egyptian and Chinese historical documents reported the use of innumerable remedies and the outcomes one could expect. In the Old Testament (estimated to range from the 15th to 4th century BC) the Book of Daniel describes what is essentially a "comparative trial" evaluating the contributions of diet to one's health.

"Then Daniel said to the steward. . . . .

"Test your servants for ten days; let us be given vegetables to eat and water to drink. Then let your appearance and the appearance of the youth who eat the King's rich food be observed by you, and according to what you see deal with your servants.

So he harkened to them in this matter, and tested them for 10 days.

At the end of ten days it was seen that they were better in appearance and fatter in flesh than all the youth who ate the King's rich food. So the steward took away their rich food and the wine they were to drink, and gave them vegetables."

Daniel 1:11-16

Thus, one sees a clinical trial of sorts to establish optimum feeding of royal disciples. Besides early comparative studies, one sees many observational studies throughout history. There are the observations of Hippocrates, a Greek physician (born 460 BC) or the teachings of Pericles who chronicled disease, treatments and outcomes. This tradition of "medical chronicles", the recording of therapies and outcomes can be traced through the centuries to the work of Consillia (14th century) who in his treatises compares cases with a disease to groups receiving an intervention, a form of a case study.

History does not only reveal recorded observations, but the applications of observation to the understanding of clinical phenomenon. The work of William Harvey, (1578-1657) physician to the King of England chronicles his observations in animals that he used to understand cardiovascular physiology and the circulation of blood in man. It was another English physician, James Lind (1747) working as a navel physician who made a seminal observation on the disease "scurvy" and then affirming his observation with a clinical trial, though one quite under powered.

Treatment	Outcome cured/number studied
Sulfuric Acid	0/2
Vinegar	0/2
Seawater	0/2
Cider	0/2
Nutmeg, garlic, cinnamon	0/2
Citrus fruit	2/2

His conclusion was that citrus fruit treated scurvy effectively.

We not only see studies evaluating therapeutic interventions, but we see an understanding of the problem of bias and the use of "blinding" to overcome bias. Louis XVI, King of France (1774) as were many in France fascinated by what in that time was referred to as "animal magnetism" – the ability of magnetism to cure disease. A commission was appointed with the American representative and discoverer of lightening as being electricity, Benjamin Franklin as its head. Dr. Franklin (an honorary title) had the foresight to have patients wear a blind and thus they did not know if magnetism was applied or not. The outcome was that there was no correlation between magnets and the effective treatment of disease. While this report received great notoriety in its day, the use of magnets as a medical treatment by "quacks" persisted throughout the 19th century in America showing that definitive studies do not always put an end to quackery.

Smallpox has been a dreaded disease for centuries. Hans Sloane, an early 18th century English physician had reported that inoculation of healthy people with puss from smallpox infected patients would prevent severe disease although with many developing the disease and some dying, James Jurin extended these observations, reporting that 5/6 died if exposed to smallpox who haven't been previously exposed to cowpox. Edward Jenner (1721) developed a method of decreasing the virulence of the cowpox and systematically inoculating a population and later reporting on the success of reducing smallpox in the population treated. These observations revolutionized the treatment of smallpox and the concept of vaccination. His use of a re-challenge of patients with smallpox to show that they are immune introduced the "rechallenge" concept into clinical medicine.

William Withering after ten years of observational studies on the use of extract from the Foxglove plant reported his results of treatment of "dropsy" what we would call heart failure today, in over 180 patients. He found the drug to be effective and by titrating the dose, recommended how to use the extract safely with reduced amounts. These studies add to our knowledge on not only the evaluation of effectiveness, but the requisite dose for effectiveness and for safety.

It is hard to envision today the mortal risk that childbirth posed in earlier times. The keen observation of the American physician Oliver Wendall Holmes reported in the book "On the Contagiousness of Puerperal Fever" (1843) that the fatal disease occurring after delivery was contagious and could be spread by attendants to the delivery. While his report caused some to change their approach, it took a more systematic study by Ignaz

Semmelweis (1818-1865) who observed as a resident in Vienna that the maternal death rate was 10-50% in the First Maternity Division of Vienna General Hospital where births were attended by physicians who performed autopsies earlier in the day as opposed to childbirths in the Second Division Ward where the mortality was 2-3% and where births were assisted by midwives. Semmelweis argued for antiseptic procedure but received no support from the senior staff in Vienna. Leaving Vienna with disapproval by his superiors. He returned to Budapest and undertook a study carefully comparing the results of antisepsis with lime as compared to standard practice, demonstrating a marked reduction in death due to sepsis. This study markedly changed the approach to surgical practice around the world. This demonstrates the power of a carefully designed clinical study.

Through not a clinical research undertaking, the experimental studies of Robert Koch (1843-1910) and the promulgation of what is called today Koch's postulates has made a lasting impression on how we look at proof of etiology. Koch postulates, constitutes a criterion designed to establish a causative relationship for a microbe and disease. His postulates have evolved into a broader concept of causality.

The postulates are:

1)The causative agent must be found with the disease.

2)One must isolate the causative agent from the disease.

3)The causative agent should transmit the disease.

4)The micro-organism (the causative agent) must be re-isolated from the re-inoculated subject.

Approaches following these postulates went a long way in requiring a scientific approach to laboratory and clinical studies.

There are many examples of careful observational studies and experimental trials in man, especially in the area of infectious disease that lead to major advances in medicine in the 19th and early 20th centuries. Gerhed Hansen (1874) believed mycobacterium leprae found in patients with leprosy was the cause of the disease. Hansen undertook a series of procedures introducing the bacillus into healthy individuals, some of whom did not know of his actions, or comprehended its significance. The concept of the requirement of patient consent for a clinical study was unfortunately not established. Hansen's actions are quite different from that of Walter Reed, a U.S. Army physician who led a research project (1901) confirming that yellow fever is transmitted by the bite of the Aedes mosquitos. However, for his study he insisted that subjects give consent before participating in the study. Reed and William Osler were strong advocates of the necessity of obtaining informed consent in clinical studies.

The 20th century saw the rapid advancement in medicine with numerous scientific advances. But many of these advances in basic science would not have been translated so effectively and rapidly if there was not a cadre of physician's primed for these advances. Abraham Flexner (1925) through the commission he headed, and its report markedly changed medical training, introducing a medical teaching program with first basic science followed by a systematic clinical instruction period rather than the prior apprentice system. His noteworthy remark that "Research can no more be divorced from medical education than can medical education be divorced from research" sounds obvious today but was not till the early part of the 20th century accepted. Even today there are medical schools that regulate research to a very limited role.

Alexander Fleming's (1925) observations with molds on plates of bacteria leading to penicillin therapy and the work of Banting and Best (1921) with insulin are just two of the major advancements we see in the early 20th century that revolutionized medical therapy and the practice of medicine. With the breakthrough in basic medical science and the clinical trial techniques available at that time, a true revolution in medicine occurred. Some of these rapid advancements were facilitated and given credence due to the work of Ronald Fisher (1920-30) in England on plant breeding where he introduced the concept of randomization techniques, blinding, and statistical testing to account for the possibility of results had occurred by chance. While Fisher's work was far removed from medicine and from clinical trials, his work had a great influence on how we design a trial and determine the reliability of its conclusions. Torall Sollman added an additional dimension to our understanding of a trial by asserting the need for controlled experiments and the utilization of a placebo, or a comparator and the importance of maintaining a blind. He was an advocate of the "blind test", determining outcome without the knowledge of the observer or the individuals being studied. One of the first areas that these concepts were applied was in the work of Nathaniel Quid

(1940's) who studied angina pectoris therapies using a "blind test" and a placebo. Interestingly, Nathaniel Quid was my first medical attending when I was a medical student in my first rotation.

The evaluation of medical therapies, how medical discoveries are made and how they are tested is quite remarkable. I have not done the field justice and have omitted many individuals who have made very important advances in disease diagnosis and therapies. Let this brief introduction serve to give the reader an overview of how our thinking has evolved and some of the issues that arise and how we now need to approach a problem in a systematic way as we proceed.

Chapter 2

Clinical Trials – An Overview

Medicine has a long history of being practiced based on observation and learnered opinion. This approach offered some diagnostic benefit and effective therapies, but advances were slow and far between. The utilization of the scientific method and experiments first in the pre-clinical and then clinical realm, especially in infectious disease led to numerous advances in the 19th century. The introduction and utilization of the clinical trial has transformed medicine from an "art" to the practice of evidence-based medicine more often than not. Fundamental to those advances has been the development of clinical research employing clinical trials.

Clinical trials have aided in the knowledge of the etiologies of disease, diagnostic procedure effectiveness and the effectiveness of a therapy for a specific condition. Clinical trials have also permitted us to gauge the safety of an intervention and the ability to weigh the benefits against the risks of a therapy or a therapeutic approach.

As we have seen in our brief review of the history of clinical research, the study of Lind on scurvy was an early clinical study. It evaluated a disease state (scurvy), evaluated a particular population (sailors), administered a series of interventions and found a possible effective intervention (citrus juice). The study had many of the characteristics of clinical trials methodology, a control or comparator group. Studies like those of Lind have evolved into trials that evaluate a medical condition, are often perspective and select a targeted population, apply an intervention, often using randomization and obtain follow up. Some clinical trialists believe a study to be called a clinical trial needs to be a perspective study comparing an intervention to a control in man. However, there are many important studies in man (clinical studies) that are retrospective and that are observational in design. A clinical study may be randomized or it may not be. A clinical study may be prospective, retrospective or a mixture of retrospective or perspective. A clinical trial may have a very well-designed hypothesis to evaluate, or it may attempt to develop an understanding of a clinical condition. In the field of cardiology one of the most important clinical studies is the Framingham Study that followed a population in Framingham, Massachusetts (and is still being carried out 50 years later). One important observation was the association of coronary artery disease and a myocardial infarction with elevated cholesterol levels. This observation has subsequently led to the introduction of important and very beneficial therapeutic agents and a significant reduction in coronary artery disease and myocardial infarction. Observational studies, comparative effectiveness studies, retrospective chart reviews all have an important place in clinical research. When Alton Ochsner looked back on his operative cases and those of his colleagues at his clinic and saw the association of smoking and lung cancer, a very significant clinical association was made. One can't randomize a population to smoking and no smoking and follow patients for 20 or 30 years to determine the casualty of smoking to lung cancer. The time frame and number required for such experiments makes them impossible, the cooperation of patients unlikely and above all the ethics of such a study design totally unacceptable.

For a clinical trial we need an hypothesis, a question or questions to try and answer. The study needs to be in man through applying clinical trial methodology to answer medical questions in animals is most appropriate and often leads to important findings. As we will see, the clinical trial needs to carefully define the population to study, needs to determine the appropriate intervention(s), its intensity, dose, frequency and needs to employ techniques to reduce bias. Measures to ensure proper randomization and blinding so the patient and researcher don't know who receives the intervention helps insure the veracity of the results.

Unquestionably, the optimum clinical trial is one that is hypothesis driven, that is randomized, that is double-blinded and that has the "power" to make a determination

that there is a high likelihood of the outcome being correctly determined and unlikely to have occurred by chance (that it is statistically significant). As we progress through our clinical research journey, we will discuss many aspects of optimizing a clinical trial to help insure the validity of our findings. But the perfect clinical trial is an impossibility, and we can only strive for the best possible design given that we deal with patients that have the right to act as they wish and that we must always be guided by the ethical practice of research.

As an example of the many conundrums in clinical research, we can only look to a trial evaluating a new therapy for heart failure. Heart failure is a very severe condition, more deadly than most cancers. Evaluating a new therapy would be best in a randomized trial with a comparator group receiving a placebo. That is not possible, since it would be unethical medical malpractice not to give all patients therapies that have proven to be effective in reducing mortality. Thus, in the field of heart failure, studies are done on top of existing effective therapies. If a therapy has properties suggesting to be effective it is possible to compare the therapy on top of established background therapy to background therapy. However, introducing a no therapy or placebo group would not be possible or acceptable medical research or acceptable medical practice. Thus, we can see how a clinical researcher faces constraints that are not faced by the basic scientist working in the pre-clinical area.

Another critical aspect of clinical research is equipoise of the investigator. If the investigator strongly believes a therapy is beneficial or harmful, it is unethical to undertake a study of that intervention. Besides being unethical, the investigator that is overly committed to a therapy may introduce biases in a study design or its execution. Equipoise is a critical component of clinical research. There are times that this poses a major problem for clinical research and while there are trial designs that try to overcome this problem ("play the winner" for example) there are serious flaws to these approaches making these research designs very problematic.

It is not so long ago that perhaps the first clinical trial utilizing randomization of an intervention vs a placebo was undertaken with thought to obtaining a statistically significant outcome (British Medical Research Council Trial – British Medical J 1948;12:769-782). Studies like these have set us on a course for the practice of evidence-based medicine. We all aspire to practice scientific truth and avoid the failings of our medical biases. But even following good clinical practice there are difficulties clinical researchers face. The medical community and society need to be accepting of the concept of therapeutic equipoise and the possibility of unexpected findings.

An early example that the medical community was not receptive to a research outcome is the difficulty that Ignaz Semmelweis faced with the results of his studies on antisepsis and the avoidance of puerperal fever and post-partum mortality. A study can be effectively carried out, but the medical community may not be prepared to accept the results. When I was initially involved in clinical cardiac electrophysiology and the technique of programmed electrical stimulation to induce susceptible patients into ventricular tachycardia and/or fibrillation, the reaction of many established physicians and members of the ethics board overseeing clinical research was outrage. Provoking a life-threatening condition in vulnerable patients was considered madness. But treating patients with therapies of dubious efficacy, untested, was readily accepted.

A clinical investigator needs to effectively communicate the need for studies, the need to proactively evaluate therapies and to explain one's approach to patients, families, and the lay public. Even with undertaking these actions, one still may face great resistance to undertaking appropriate and important clinical research.

Clinical research is limited by the way we ask the research question, the technologies we have available to evaluate outcomes and the methods for research outcome evaluation. We are also limited by our own capabilities to utilize the existing technologies. There is a learning process (a learning curve) that is involved with many of the techniques we use in medicine and that must be considered in evaluating the research we produce. The surgical technique, the medical intervention, the methods we use to assess an intervention often poses a very steep learning process, that can considerably impact the results of a study. The "learning curve" must be taken into consideration in the design of a clinical study, and the studies assessment. It is also important to take into consideration when the technique is introduced into clinical practice. A novel technique may selectively recruit a different population than an established approach.

Different areas of research have different established approaches to diagnosis and treatment and at times differing approaches to the methods of undertaking clinical research. Perhaps this is most evident in the development of pharmaceutical agents where clinical studies are classified as Phase I, II, III & IV.

Phase I studies are first in man studies, usually with the intent to evaluate the pharmacokinetics of a drug. They are small studies usually involving 6-12 patients in a group. Sometimes they are undertaken to determine safety, other times to assess a dose that causes an easily determined outcome such as BP or QT interval effect on the ECG. The studies are usually performed in normal's. But some drugs are too toxic to be given to normal patients and the studies are performed in patients at the doses intended for treatment. This is often the case with oncology therapies.

Phase II studies are often aimed to determine optimum dose, dose finding studies, or studies aimed at an early determination of efficacy, such as blood pressure lowering, an easily measured endpoint. These studies are done in patients, are small in number (50-200 patients) and are often done at a single center.

Phase III studies are often planned as the definitive studies in a drug development program. The studies are appropriately powered to be of a size likely to yield statistically significant results to demonstrate that the drug is effective. The studies are usually multi-centered and often look to obtain a natural history outcome (hospitalization, death) as opposed to earlier phase II studies with physiologic endpoints not assessing natural history outcomes. Since the studies usually follow patients for 1-2 years, the comparator is usually standard therapy since prolonged administration of a placebo is not acceptable.

Phase IV studies are by definition performed after the new drug application has been submitted to FDA. They may be additional large outcome studies, they may be in differing populations, or in patients with a somewhat different underlying condition or co-morbidity as in patients with another underlying disease such as renal dysfunction. The Phase IV studies may be aimed at evaluating drug – drug interactions, or metabolism in select populations. Additionally, Phase IV studies may be done for a marketing purpose, establishing the comparative effectiveness of the drug as compared to a competing product. While done for marketing purposes, these studies may be very useful to a clinician trying to decide in which patient and when to use the drug. Phase IV studies can help position a drug in a physician's therapeutic armamentarium. In the European Union (EU) to market a drug it must be compared to its major competitor. This is not the case in the U.S. making comparative assessment more difficult.

Pharmaceutical studies are carried out under an investigational new drug application (IND). A study carried out after a New Drug Application submission to FDA is a Phase IV study. A Phase IV study can be carried out after the drug is marketed, but still under the initial IND. If a drug is studied for a new indication, a new IND is needed and the new indication will need to be applied for through an NDA. A drug lowering BP indicated for hypertension, may be useful in heart failure treatment. Even if approved for hypertension, to study its use in heart failure requires a new IND and to obtain the indication in the product label, a new NDA submitted to FDA for review and possible approval would be needed for marketing the drug for this indication.

Ethics

Whether it be a study evaluating a new surgical technique, a new drug, or a method of disease diagnosis, the study will need to be ethically designed and executed under the approval of an investigational review board (ethical review board or IRB). That a study is ethical first requires that it is scientifically justified, that it has a reasonable chance of success and that the investigators are qualified to execute the study. A study too small in size, even if its goals are scientifically sound, is an unethical study, putting the patients or volunteers at risk for a limited scientific benefit. A small study can be performed ethically if it is a pilot study, evaluating the feasibility of the study plan or to train the staff on procedures that would be needed for a larger, definitive trial. Convention has it that a study should have an 80% probability of demonstrating a significant effect at the statistical level of $p < 0.05$, thus affording a 1 in 20 chance of a false positive outcome. This number needed to study is determined by the estimates of effect size and the probability of success the investigators have accepted. This is obtained in a power calculation.

Even with a reasonable statistical chance of success and a reasonable scientific justification of the study, a clinical trial must treat its patients ethically. There is an unfortunate history of scientifically sound, but unethical studies that have led to a need for investigators to understand accepted ethical standards for research.

Studies through the centuries invariably entered patients in trials without the patient's consent, without the patient having an understanding of the potential risks and benefits when taking part in a study. William Osler and Walter Reid were the early exceptions in the 19th century, arguing for obtaining a patient's consent to include them in a study.

Far more sinister were the numerous experiments performed in Nazi Germany in support of Nazi theories of eugenics and "racial superiority". Over the course of the Nazi regimen (1933-1945) physicians and scientists went beyond eugenics and racial studies in using concentration camp prisoners (Jews, Roma, homosexuals, disabled, diseased or medically infirm German citizens) to undertake experiments sometimes thought to benefit the military in its performance of missions, in tolerating inhospitable clients and in developing improved killing strategies. In the concentration camp at Dachau the German air force undertook studies freezing helpless prisoners, exposing them to low oxygen saturation and high-pressures, unimaginable torture; to possibly improve functioning of air force pilots. Perhaps most infamous are the experiments of "doctor" Joseph Mengele who performed horrific experiments on twins, sterilizing them, torturing them with surgeries to damage organs and to alter their physiology to determine these actions on survival. Innocent prisoners, or those accused of opposition to the Nazi government were infected with disease and tested to see if sulfonamide or other therapies would be effective. People were given "sea water" at various saline concentrations to determine at what concentration life could be sustained. Experiments were conducted at Buchenwald to investigate the effect of poisons. Some were left to die in an agonizing pain and others killed immediately to perform autopsies to obtain an understanding of the pathotoxicologic effects of these agents. There were bone, muscle and nerve transplantation experiments, head injury experiments, malaria experiments, hepatic injury experiments, mustard gas experiments, blood coagulation experiments and electroshock experiments all for the most part leading to agonizing deaths. These experiments are inconceivable, inhumane undertakings that need to be known by all and condemned by all involved in clinical research, but especially by physicians who have sworn an oath to alleviate suffering and cure disease. These horrific acts against mankind led to the Nuremberg Code in 1947 that began a more formalized process of establishing ethical standards in clinical research (The Nuremberg Code, available at: http/www.hhs.gov/ohrp/archive/nurcode.html). The code outlines ethical standards for clinical research, mandating informed and willing consent of participants.

In 1932, 600 African Americans in Macon County Alabama at Tuskegee University entered a study sponsored by the US Public Health Service. The study consisted of 399 men with latent syphilis and 201 who were not infected. The patients were offered free medical care for study participation, but in fact were not given state of the art therapy as it became available. This was done to study the natural history of the disease. Not informing patients of the risks and not administering possibly effective treatment was unacceptable.

In 1956 a study began at the Willowbrook State School in Staten Island, NY to understand the transmission of hepatitis, a common disease suffered by most children at the school. The school specialized in care for children with mental retardation. The studies were undertaken to understand how hepatitis was spread, how to prevent the disease and what viruses caused the disease. Students were given the hepatitis virus believed to be in fecal samples from diseased children and the children were subsequently followed. No consent was obtained from parents, no student was informed of the study and no parent was informed of the risks involved.

In both of these landmark examples of ethical lapses, physicians justified their actions on the basis of the need to understand how the disease progressed, untreated and in the Willowbrook Study to understand the disease transmission. These arguments do not justify letting syphilis go untreated and guaranteeing all children a hepatitis infection and its irreversible squali.

Clinical experiments like these led to the World Medical Association studying the issue and then promulgating the Declaration of Helsinki (http://www.net/en/30publicatioons/10policies/3/index.html). This comprehensive statement of the approach to the ethical undertaking of clinical research should be read by all those involved in clinical research. The Congress of the United States authorized a study on clinical research which was circulated as the

Belmont Report in 1979. Though never formally adapted by the U.S. Congress as law, the report serves as the basis of ethical clinical research standards for the Department of Health and Human Services and that of the National Institute of Health (NIH).

Physicians and all perspective clinical researchers should take the time to familiarize themselves with some of the key examples of clinical research gone awry. One should read the Declaration of Helsinki and the Belmont Report, as well as participating in ethics training, a requirement by all IRB's to undertake clinical research. Ethical training can be obtained through the NIH (https://www.bioethics.nih.gov) or through CITI services at https://about.citiprogram.org. CITI offers a very reasonably priced basic introduction to clinical ethics through an online module that can be updated yearly to remain in IRB compliance.

Ethics training must involve an understanding of conflict of interests, the requirements of informed consent (which will be covered in the IRB chapter), the need to maintain patient privacy and the issues involved in the early termination of a research study. Many of these issues may not be as simple as they first appear.

Financial relationships can often pose a conflict of interest. The disclosure of a potential or real conflict of interest is important. But disclosure alone does not annul a potential conflict. In fact, all investigators have conflicts of interest. Most investigators receive financial support for undertaking clinical studies. One advances one's scientific career through research and positive studies do this so much more effectively than negative studies. The best work is often done by investigators who are motivated by potential financial gain. The development of a device or drug is usually the principal motivation driving the clinical research process. It's a difficult balance needing oversight at academic institutions, companies and IRB's, but most important the physician researcher scientist must be guided by moral principles. Falsifying research, "cutting corners", hiding non-supporting findings is wrong, can place the investigator in legal jeopardy and harm patients. Bias can lead to false findings, pressure to falsify data and the propagation of misinformation that eventually and invariably will be exposed. The investigator, that is financially conflicted, however, should not be excluded from clinical research. The investigator researching his idea, being the advocate of a drug or device is perhaps the best way to make progress. By adhering to good clinical methods and practices, the validity of the results will be more likely. The lack of good methodologies, the lack of disclosure, promulgating misinformation and deceitful practices will always come to be revealed with severe consequences. A positive example is Michael Mirowski's tenacity in developing and studying the utility of the implantable defibrillator. His work is an excellent example of the benefits coming from someone who is an inventor, investigator, advocating for his invention and studying its effectiveness. Without his tireless efforts, the great benefits derived from this medical device may have been missed.

Most clinical trials, drugs and device studies offer benefits and come with associated risks. These potential benefits and risks need to be appropriately verified during clinical trials and after the therapy's approval. A study that is blinded and multi-centered usually has a data safety monitoring board (DSMB) overseeing the project. During the course of a study, one may see a trend towards adversity. It is possible that the outcome of the study may be negative, and the adverse outcome may reach statistical significance. Stopping a study prematurely may yield a situation where the outcome is in question. However, failing to stop the study may lead to patient harm. An example is the University Group Diabetes Studies in Type II diabetes that were stopped early. After the study was stopped and reported some believed that oral hypoglycemic agents cause adverse cardiovascular outcomes and the efficacy and safety of this class of drugs was not established. Stopping a study is a very difficult decisions that a DSMB has to consider that can have profound, lasting consequences.

Additional Ethical Questions

There are many other areas where ethical questions may arise. An investigator may change position, lose interest in a study or find the study results to be negative. Often this leads to abandonment of the project. But patients or volunteers took risks being involved in the study and for this reason the information obtained should be analyzed and published. Not publishing the results of a negative study may lead to the study or a similar one being repeated, a waste of resources and placing others at risk. Negative studies, studies with disagreeable results should be published. Incomplete studies that are not to be finished should be analyzed and if possible, an abstract of the work reported. Studies performed with pharmaceutical industry support may yield results that are negative or with findings not pleasing to the sponsor. An investigator needs to give the sponsor appropriate warning and not attack the product, but complete reporting of the study outcome is imperative for medical knowledge and respects the risk patients took to be in the study. Perhaps the study design was flawed, or excessive numbers of patients were lost to follow up. These problems can be pointed out, but one should strive to report the study finding along with its failings.

We are in a time where excessive actions are at times taken in the name of ethics. To publish a study if one is studying a drug or device, the investigator must register a study in advance in a public database (ClinicalTrials.gov is often employed). However, there are reasons to want to keep knowledge of a trial away from device or pharmaceutical company competitors. This is ethical and unfortunately is very difficult, often impossible. Listing of studies to prevent suppression of publication (which is unethical) could be prevented by IRB's, the government through FDA, or through interventions by research administrators at academic institutions. There are better approaches than forcing all trials to be listed publicly. One also sees excessive involvement of Journal staff in the selection of authors. An individual may have contributed to a project but worked minimally on it. Should that person be left off as an author of the study? A head of a department or institute could have made the study financially possible, made important design suggestions and permitted the other investigators to allocate time to execute the study; should the person making the study possible be left off authorship? It appears that the actual daily work of carrying out the study is being given more value at times than the idea of conceiving the study or making the project financially possible.

International multi-center studies are more often than not utilized when large clinical trials are required because more patients can be recruited, the trials costs are often less outside the U.S. and competing therapies far fewer. However, all these advantages also have ethical and operational difficulties associated. One needs to ask are the inducements to participate in the study excessive. Is the offer of a bone marrow transplant for someone who needs it such a powerful inducement in Malaysia compared to the U.S., as to unduly influence participants to take risks they would not otherwise take? Is medical care similar at each site? Is background therapy very different from country to country and thus can influence study outcome. A study can compensate by offering the same standard of care to all participants, but will that be continued after the study is complete? Perhaps it is better to provide the best medical care possible at least during the study, offering the patients potentially better outcomes than they would otherwise have available. It is inappropriate to ask a sponsor of a study to pay indefinitely for care the patients would not otherwise receive in their country. But to stop optimum medical care is also unethical. The most problematic aspect of international studies may not be ethical questions but the difference in the understanding of disease states and the practice of medicine. An example is the study of spironolactone in patients with heart failure with preserved ejection fraction. The overall study was negative, but the results were positive when looking at the results obtained in the U.S. and Western Europe. What constitutes heart failure with preserved ejection fraction in Russia and Eastern Europe may be very different than in the U.S. or the financial incentives to randomize patients so attractive in these countries as to cause recruitment of ineligible patients.

Patient Confidentiality

It can be very detrimental for a patients to have his or her medical information, or disease they are experiencing made public. Medical history is a very private subject to be appropriately held in confidence. However, we have gone too far in protecting patient confidentiality. The process developed to maintain confidentiality is excessive, often interfering with obtaining important information. Medical outcomes of patients is often difficult to obtain. Initiating studies without background information on potential patient can compromise a study. Excessive medical confidentiality can make recruitment difficult. Using de-identified patient information should be simple and facilitated. Putting "road-blocks" in the way of carrying out clinical research is itself unethical and undercuts the common good. Unfortunately, these are the rules we need to deal with. Investigators must work with the information available and try to inform hospital administrators, IRB's, and policy makers the difficulties in initiating and conducting clinical research and the improvements that can be made to facilitate the undertaking of clinical research.

Chapter 3. The Research Trial

To undertake a research trial one needs to formulate a research question and create a research protocol. To accomplish these goals one needs to perform several critical steps to develop an appropriate research trial that can answer a research question. There are many essential issues, sample size determination, populations to be studied, primary and secondary endpoints to select. Each of these aspects of the research trial will be discussed.

The Research Question

What first must be determined is what we want to study and what is the primary research question we want to ask. It's never acceptable to ask a general question such as what causes heart disease or what causes cancer. They are admirable questions to pose but do not help in creating a framework for a successful investigation. It is essential to be as focused and specific as possible in posing the question. This enables the investigator to develop research methods and outcome variables that can be measured and thus address the research question.

One must define the area being studied, the issues involved, the endpoints to be assessed, the disease to be studied, the stage of the disease, the makeup of the population to be studied, and the duration of study.

Question Selection:

One's interest and resources should play a major factor in

selecting the research question. What is the significance of the study? Does one have the resources to undertake the study and carry it out to fruition? A study that does not have a significant impact on public health, scientific knowledge or economic consideration should probably not be undertaken. Starting a study knowing you don't have the resources to complete the project is a waste of your time and unethical to those participating in the study. It is wrong to undertake a study that is of no or little interest to the medical community or yourself, just to be involved in a study. Studies, even the simplest, take a lot of effort to complete and utilize a lot of resources that could be expended on more important questions. One should not undertake a study because you have developed a questionnaire or know a statistical technique, just to have a result that can be published. Choose a study that asks a useful question, that has import. Then think about the most important outcome that can be successfully and effectively measured and identify the outcome as the primary measure. It is usually best to have a single primary outcome, but some studies may be successfully executed with more than one primary outcome if the study is appropriately powered for the multiple primary outcomes. It is best to have an outcome variable that sheds light on the mechanism underlying the benefit or risk of the intervention. All-cause mortality may not be as useful as a disease specific mortality (though identifying a disease specific mortality can be problematic). If one is studying the benefits of an anti-arrhythmic therapy all-cause mortality as an outcome is not as informative as cardiac mortality or arrhythmia caused mortality, but the type of mortality may be difficult to determine. A patient can be suddenly stricken with chest pain and then expire. Was the death an acute MI or an arrhythmia causing hypotension, decreased cardiac output and subsequently ischemia that caused death? The cause of death can be difficult to categorize. One may want to use sudden death as the endpoint. Differentiating cardiac mortality from sudden cardiac death mortality? If the death is defined as sudden death cardiac, what is the timeframe of sudden (minutes, hours, or 24 hours, as some studies have employed). These are important issues when developing the primary research question. All-cause mortality is informative because the endpoint encompasses all mechanism underlying mortality and can be readily determined. An anti-arrhythmic agent can reduce arrhythmias but can also enhance arrhythmias and mortality. Thus, reporting both arrhythmias associated mortality and all-cause mortality is appropriate.

Another important issue in considering the research question is can the question be answered or is the study likely to fail. Always phrase the question so it has an outcome that can be measured and concerns a question that can be answered.

If one can't ascertain the endpoint, it is likely that the research question can't be answered. It is best to present the research question as a hypothesis. By doing this the investigator's equipoise is maintained with an alternative null hypothesis postulated. One can state a hypothesis as to risk of a disease, risk of an outcome, the benefit of an intervention (procedure or therapy), or the possibility of equivalence or non-inferiority.

Besides the primary question, there are often additional questions to be asked. It is important to aim to obtain the maximum information from a study. While survival is important, understanding the cause of the disease is also important. The disease duration, the need for hospitalization, the ability of a patient to work, the need for additional therapies, the patient's residual disability; are all important considerations. One powers a study for the primary outcome. Asking multiple secondary questions that the study can't possibly answer with any probability of success is inappropriate. Thus, when powering a study, one needs to account for the sample size needed for the secondary endpoints as well, if one intends for those secondary outcomes to be addressed. A study with a primary endpoint often has two or three secondary questions poised. More than two or three secondary questions usually can't be reasonably answered with any reasonable probability and thus should not be considered. If there are critical secondary questions to address, increasing the number of patients may be needed for the possibility of success.

The response variable may be different among the study endpoints. One may have as the primary endpoint the reduction in blood pressure, a continuous variable and a secondary endpoint, the development of a myocardial infarction or heart failure, categorical variables.

Secondary Question:

A secondary question may be related to the primary outcome in a select group of the population. Gender is a secondary question often asked. Does a drug or is a procedure effective in both men and women? Ethnicity can be an important consideration since ethnicity can be a way (though imperfect) in asserting genetic considerations in the outcome of the primary response variable. Ethnicity – Asian, African American, Caucasian, may suggest different mechanisms of disease, immunologic response, or metabolic pathway of drug metabolism and inactivation. However, patients' self-identification may be inaccurate and genetic considerations and ethnicity may not be correlated. While people of Asian decent may metabolize a drug differently, less effectively, there is a considerable variability within groups. Still the characterization of the primary response variables outcome in distinct ethnic groups, age, stages of disease or disease severity may be very informative. A secondary question may be a broader evaluation of an outcome. Sudden death may be the primary outcome and one may ask a secondary question of all-cause mortality.

Adversity

It may be a goal of a clinical investigator to determine the safety of a procedure or a treatment. While Phase III pharmaceutical studies are usually undertaken primarily to determine drug efficacy, understanding the body's response to prolonged therapy is important safety outcome. A prolonged evaluation of safety is often obtained in a Phase III or Phase IV clinical trial. However, designing a trial specifically to determine an adverse outcome has significant ethical limitations. A trial for the express purpose of determining toxicity is usually not undertaken. That does not preclude the assessment of a risk of prolonged treatment and thus the determination of a risk/benefit ratio. If one is performing a comparative study of two antibiotics one can have the hypothesis that Drug A is better than Drug B and that Drug A is safer than Drug B, though both may be effective therapies. Most often the study of a therapeutic is not powered statistically to determine adversity, but rather a toxicity evaluation is observational in nature. In drug development trials this lack of power for toxicity assessment poses limitations. Phase I trials have a couple of dozen patients. A toxicity that occurs 1 out of 100 exposures will probably not be seen. Phase II studies with a couple of hundred patients is also unlikely to reveal a toxicity even with a high frequency of 1 in 100 exposures. However, in Phase III studies 1 in 100 exposures frequency of toxicity is likely to be seen, although possibly not identified as definitely drug related. If the incidence was 1/1000, only a couple of instances would be reported in a Phase III program of 3,000 to 5,000 patients. This lack of sensitivity can result in drugs with a somewhat frequent toxicity being approved and only picked up post marketing. This can extend even to Phase IV trials with the toxicity not identified. The toxicity may only be identified after more extensive clinical exposure during drug marketing when the exposure reaches 10, 20 or 50 thousand patients.

Specificity of the Research Question

It is most useful to be as precise with the primary and

secondary research question(s). The research question of whether Drug A is better than placebo is a standard question, but it really does not evaluate what the investigator or the research community is hoping to obtain from the study. It would be far better to ask if Drug A, at a specific dose is significantly better than a placebo in a disease of a given severity over a specified duration of administration in a particular population. Stating the research hypothesis in this detailed fashion can be very helpful in the planning of the research trial. However, such a detailed hypothesis makes the results less generalizable. One may want to know the dose of the drug to initiate and then how to be titrated the therapy. One may want to apply the drug to a broader spectrum of the disease with a more variable duration of therapy. Being overly precise may have drawbacks as does being too non-specific in specifying the research question. A balance needs to be found between being too general and being overly specific.

The Research Protocol

The clinical trial protocol is the backbone of any research project. It is so to speak the blueprint of the trial, its design and exactly how it will be undertaken, completed, and analyzed. The title states the subject and purpose of the research project. This is followed by an introduction that provides a background about the research question, what is known in the literature, and the significance of undertaking the project. The introduction is followed by a statement of objectives. The primary research question is re-stated with the relevant response variable(s) followed by the secondary research variables to be ascertained. The secondary response variables cover the subgroup analysis proposed to answer the secondary research question(s).

A statement of the study design follows. Is it a parallel or crossover study, blinded or not, and for what duration? Defining the study population is most important and this is done by a listing of the study inclusion criteria and the exclusion criteria for eliminating patients from recruitment. The size of the study is a very important consideration. It needs to be described along with the "power" calculation with its assumptions justifying the sample size.

Next the procedures to carry out the study needs to be explained in detail. How is the screening and informed consent process carried out. The baseline visit, what measurements will be made, their frequency, the subsequent study visits, procedures to be undertaken and what follow up planned. The intervention being studied needs to be described and how it will be administered. Will all subjects receive the intervention? Is it given to a single group? Is there a comparator? Is this done by randomization? What is the randomization method? How will compliance with the intervention be determined? Then one needs to explain the way the outcome(s) or response variables are obtained. Is the staff trained to be consistent and not bias the study? What are the data collection methods and what quality control procedures are to be utilized by study management?

Some protocols will be simple studies done at a single site, by a single investigator. In a multi-center, multiple investigator study a data safety monitoring board and statistical evaluation group are often needed. Larger trials have a management group involved, with a detailed description of its operation. One needs to specify training required, data collection and quality control methods as well as procedures for data analysis. How will the data be stored and how and when will it be analyzed? What statistical methods are planned and why? How will the investigators deal with lost data, patients lost to follow up and missing test data? These issues must be pre-specified in the protocol. Will there be an interim analysis? Is the patient's safety surveilled by a data safety monitoring committee (DSMB)? Are the interim analyses accounted for in the statistical plan, allowing for a loss of power with multiple interim analysis? The multiple testing for significance does affect sample size. There is a need to mention procedures for study termination and when it should be considered. If the study is found to cause harm before all patients are randomized, what will happen? What is the criteria for harm? If the study is found to be futile to continue since it will never reveal a statistically significant outcome, will the study be stopped? What is the criteria for futility?

Operation of the study should be clearly described in an operations section. Who runs the study and who is responsible for reporting to the IRB? If a drug or device is involved, who is to report outcomes to the FDA, especially adversities encountered. Who handles the statistical analysis, the quality control and data management? Who is going to write up and report the study as a publication in a scientific journal? Who will report the findings to the study investigators, the study participants and to those funding the study? What laboratories will be used, a laboratory at each site or a central laboratory? How will samples be sent to a central lab? How will samples be stored and with what precautions. What are the reference laboratory range for normal and abnormal test results (often presented in a protocol appendix)? In the protocol or in an Appendix the management team of the study should be listed, the members of a data monitoring committee and those involved in the statistical analysis and on the study's executive committee should be identified.

A protocol should touch on all the enumerated considerations mentioned. The protocol also needs to be succinct and readable, to be read by each investigator and their staff. All those involved in this study need to have a complete overview of the study for a successful outcome. The protocol is the operation manual for those executing the study. But the protocol is also the basis on which the IRB evaluates the study. It is the document that the informed consent is derived. If the study is part of a drug development program the protocol is what the FDA bases its evaluation of the study. Thus, the protocol is a most critical document.

The protocol also contains a model consent which is informative to potential investigators, and for FDA to evaluate the study. The model consent is often modified by individual IRB's and/or the FDA. It is not the final consent used at each investigative site, but a starting framework of what the final consent will look like. The consent form will be discussed in a subsequent chapter. Additionally, the study protocol is accompanied by an Investigator

Brochure (IB). This is required for drug and device studies. When the protocol is accompanied with an IB the protocol may be less descriptive in some of the sections mentioned, especially the background of the study, preliminary studies, previous studies, and experience with studies in other countries. All these topics can be covered in greater detail in the IB. Still enough information is needed in the protocol such that all personnel participating in the study are adequately informed without reading the IB.

Choosing the Research Question: Example

COVID-19 has created a considerable need for effective therapies and over 6,000 clinical trials were conducted in the U.S. in 2019-20. One area of considerable need has been for therapeutics that modify and/or shorten the disease course or reduce the adversities of hospitalization, intubation and death that results from the COVID infection. Early on old drugs that had in vitro anti-viral action such as hydroxychloroquine and ivermectin were of interest to evaluate clinically. Especially before the vaccines were available there was an urgent need for this evaluation and this need has continued. Unfortunatcly, politicians first "poisoned the well" and then so many studies were poorly conceived and undertaken that we remain two years into the pandemic often without good evidence in these areas.

As discussed in this chapter, first it is necessary to understand the condition being studied. COVID is initially a respiratory disease where a virus enters the body, infects the lungs, replicates in massive numbers and cause an immunologic mediated mobilization of the body's defenses. Lung function may become severely impaired, but the catastrophic adverse effects are due to the body's immunologic reaction to the virus and the ensuing "cytokine storm" that may severely injure or kill the host. So, with this understanding, it is more likely that an anti-viral agent may be effective in the early stage of disease. Unfortunately, so many studies target patients in hospital with immunologic pathophysiology. Why because in hospital studies during a pandemic are easier to recruit patients. The urgency for a late effective treatment to avoid bad outcomes is pressing and thus in-hospital studies are most frequently undertaken. Many of the early COVID studies were not randomized and did not have a control group. The old, misguided belief that in extreme circumstances a randomized study can't be performed in such a serious disease ethically is just not correct. Offering patients standard alternative therapy is fine, especially since many believe hydroxychloroquine or ivermectin may be harmful. Equipoise does exist for most investigators. Observational, retrospective and non-controlled studies can be initially useful as a starting point, especially with unknown agents for a given indication especially to obtain information for a starting dose or potential toxicities to be on the lookout for their occurrence. Hydroxychloroquine and invenectum are very well characterized agents although the optimum dose for COVID was unknown (if there is one). Uncontrolled, observational studies will not be helpful in establishing an optimum dose for drug efficacy. This is exactly what happened with conflicting uncontrolled studies that have left knowledge of these agents' efficacy, the correct dose and when to employ them unknown for over two years in the pandemic. The pandemic took us back a century or two in more ways than is currently understood. So much for an understanding of the scientific method and clinical trials methodology was not appropriately applied. Perhaps we all can agree that the U.S. does not have an effective system for determining drug efficacy in emergency situations for re-purposed agents. A more organized process that can be rapidly initiated is urgently needed.

The research question should have been: Does the agent _______________ at dose X, given ________ hours after the onset of COVID symptoms to patients not hospitalized, reduce the combined endpoint of duration of symptoms, hospitalization, ICU administration, dialysis, intubation and death as compared to patients receiving placebo therapy. Placebo therapy would be administered on top of standard of care therapy if placebo was felt to be unethical. In fact there was no out of hospital initiated therapy sanctioned for over a year.

We have seen inadequate studies initially on potential repurposed therapies. Instead we saw studies focused on the evaluation of very costly new anti-viral's with potential serious side effects. We have also seen extensive development programs for vaccines and novel anti-viral's leading to emergency use authorizations initially with inadequate follow up with inadequate pharmacovigilance and generalizations to sub-groups tested in insufficient numbers for far too short a duration. We have also seen a disregard for the selection of potential therapies based on the individual patient's risk benefit ratio for a specific therapy. Seeing the approval of vaccines for the young without adequately powered trials and without taking into consideration the risk vs. benefit in these special populations is unfortunate.

Chapter 4.

Measurements of Outcome and Risk

Often a research study may be undertaken to determine an outcome. The hypothesis of the study should thus contain an outcome measure. The outcome measure can be continuous or categorical. An example of a continuous variable is blood pressure, while the most definitive categorical variable is death. A study may have multiple secondary variables and they can be categorical or continuous. For example, a study can have as its primary variable a lowering of blood pressure, while the secondary variable could be side effect free or death, both categorical variables. The use of a continuous variable often reduces the sample size needed for statistical power, an advantage. However, a categorical natural history endpoint is often most important, such as death due to ineffective blood pressure control. The reduction in death would require a far larger number to study but would make a very significant statement on the therapeutic intervention.

Measurement of Outcome

Response variables may differ a great deal, from death to economic impact, from adverse events to quality of life. A response variable can vary from disease incidence to a biomarker or even a laboratory test results. In designing a measurement of outcome, the appropriate characteristics of a variable is that it relates to the stated hypothesis and will yield a clear result, enabling the investigator to state clearly if the hypothesis is accepted or if indeed the null hypothesis is correct, that the outcome does not support the hypothesis. It is unfortunate if the response variable does not completely encompass the outcome being measured resulting in the investigator unable to adequately evaluate the study's hypothesis. When this happens, it is regrettable. However, it may not be possible to measure a response variable that encompasses the entire effect one is attempting to measure. It is also important to choose a response variable that is clinically significant with "cut offs" that are clinically meaningful. A reduction in blood pressure of 2 mmHg may be statistically significant in a study, but a 2mm reduction in blood pressure in a patient with a 110 mm diastolic BP resulting in a BP of 108 would not be considered clinically significant. A reduction in a rash by 10% in a dermatologic study may meet a study defined goal, but would a patient be satisfied with a 10% reduction in their skin risk? We are usually pooling results and thus a mean reduction of 10% may be associated with a clinically satisfactory reduction in the rash, as well a 2mm mean reduction in BP. This might be dependent on the etiology of the rash being treated with some responding to the therapy dramatically and others with a different rash etiology, responding minimally or not at all. This speaks to the need to attempt to make the condition being studied as homogenous as possible. The downside is that a very homogenous population or a very homogenous condition may not be generalizable to the entire population with the condition. Not understanding critical facets of the condition being treated or characteristics of the study population increasing effectiveness of treatment results in not knowing the patients who will respond. The stage of the disease, an understanding of the pathophysiology involved and knowledge of who may respond are important factors in the selection of the appropriate outcome measurements that will provide informative results.

Multiple measures of a response variable may lead to false positive results, since by chance one may stumble on a statistically significant positive outcome. Thus, evaluating the significance of a response variable requires an adequate sample size and the avoidance of multiple testing for significance since repeated tests can dramatically reduce the power of a study – resulting I an outcome by chance. This danger of multiple testing leading to a chance significant outcome is especially prevalent with multiple secondary endpoints. Secondary endpoints can be informative since they often give insight to mechanistic questions, or they identify other important variables associated with outcome. In a blood pressure study a significant lowering of blood pressure by a mean of 5 mmHg or greater by an agent may be an important metric. However, secondary endpoints related to mental acuity, side effects and tolerability are also important questions. A potent agent that has more side effects that is not well tolerated or causes substantial confusion would be useful clinically to know and may significantly change one's assessment of the therapy. It is important to pre specify endpoints both the primary and secondary. If an outcome is not pre specified it may permit investigator bias or be the result of chance. Having multiple secondary endpoints, beyond 2-3 may so reduce power and result in findings that are not significant, leading to a false negative outcome. Pre specifying endpoints avoids misleading or incorrect observations that are obtained by data dredging. However, at times underpowered results, or results that were not pre specified, may still be of value as hypothesis generating. These results are not determinative. As long as the results are understood to be preliminary, needing confirmation in a future study they can be useful observations.

To this point we have been focused on an outcome of a response variable. However, in certain circumstances it may be more important to measure the frequency of outcome. The number of episodes of ventricular tachycardia in a 24-hour period is a useful indication of risk for sudden death, perhaps more than a single short run of VT. The reduction in the frequency of epileptic seizure is an important clinical measure. Often in medicine we can't reduce the adverse variable incidence to zero, but we can reduce it to a more manageable frequency. Administration of an anti-arrhythmic to patients with an implantable defibrillator is done to decrease arrhythmias that may trigger a shock and thus reduce the incidence of shocks which can be harmful. Drugs are unfortunately not 100% effective but a marked reduction in device shocks has been shown to reduce the development of heart failure. Thus in a study the frequency of shocks may be a far more important endpoint than time to first shock or just counting any shock as a failure.

A study may not employ a single response variable but may

combine response variables into a group, a composite. It is best that the composite endpoint reflects an underlying mechanism such as embolization combined with a blood clotting marker (D-dimer) The composite endpoint should not consist of unrelated outcomes. In a number of important trials in the cardiology field the composite of death, myocardial infarction, hospitalization and stroke are combined. This sort of combination aids the investigator statistically by dealing with the problem of censoring when a patient dies. With the combined endpoint if the patient dies the outcome is counted, if the patient has an MI or stroke, an event is counted. Death as a single endpoint which could also be informative and can be employed alone as a secondary one, but as the primary endpoint would require a much larger study. Unfortunately, often studies employ composite endpoints of varying degrees of clinical importance. Death, MI, hospitalization and positive cardiac enzymes are frequently combined. While cardiac enzymes are often employed to diagnose a myocardial infarction, we know that an enzyme release can follow a brief period of coronary occlusion or after an obstruction to the coronary vessel(s) is relieved but before the heart muscle is permanently damaged. If the primary composite endpoint is death, MI, hospitalization and enzyme release but most of the differences in outcome between groups is due to enzyme release the importance of the study outcome may be substantially reduced. What is driving the study results needs to be known and the endpoints impact on the clinical significance of the study results recognized. A study conclusion driven by a minor outcome in the composite endpoint to the casual reader of the study may be very misleading. It may be that the difference in the primary variable showed a 23% risk reduction at $p<0.0001$ all due to a measurement of a less important component (enzyme elevation in this example).

It can also be problematic when the composite variables are not moving in the same direction or showing the same magnitude of effect. Death and hospitalization may be benefited, but a reduction in stroke is not. What would that mean if stroke increases while the other components of the composite decreases? Consistency of the response is an important metric. If the endpoints of CV death and stroke diverge, this may be an important observation suggesting differences in pathophysiologic response to therapy between the cardiac and brain vasculature. While composite endpoints can help deal with the issue of death that censors the ability to count other variables, composite endpoints pose their share of issues in trial interpretation. When one combines in a composite outcome variables including discordant variables such as toxicity (bleeding) with outcome variables of death and MI occurrence one can end up with confusing results. An example could be less bleeding, but an increase in death and MI, The clinical value of such a combined result would be perplexing. Would the increase in bleeding reduce the significance of the outcome? Is death or MI on the same level of a bleed (especially a minor or moderately severe bleed)?

Measurement of Risk

The proportion of previously unaffected individuals who acquire a disease is a risk. There can be absolute risk in which the time frame is specified or there can be relative risk, the risk of one group compared to another. One can look at the ratio of risk;

$$\frac{\text{Disease risk in exposed to a disease}}{\text{Disease risk in the non-exposed}}$$

One can determine the difference in risk or incidence of disease as:

Disease risk in exposed – disease risk in the non-exposed

We can ask how much of a risk is attributed to a given exposure. This is the attributable risk and can be a very useful metric. The risk that may be just associated with the exposure or there may be causality. We can ask how much of the risk of disease can be assigned as contributory. If we reduce or remove the risk how much of the disease can be eliminated? We can determine the attributable risk of the exposed group:

Incidence in exposed group – incidence in non-exposed group

One can ask what proportion of risk in exposed individuals is due to disease exposure and show the attributed risk as a proportion of the total incidence in the exposed group that is attributable to the exposure by:

$$\frac{\text{Incidence in exposed group} - \text{incidence in non-exposed group}}{\text{Incidence in exposed group}}$$

The incidence can be defined as the fraction of individuals who develop a condition over a defined period (often a year). Prevalence is defined as the overall number with a given condition.

One can also determine the risk of an entire population not just those exposed:

Incidence of disease in total population – Incidence in the non-exposed
(Background risk)

Besides attributable risk there is the concept of relative risk:

$$\frac{\text{Risk in exposed}}{\text{Risk in non-exposed}}$$

This gives us the probability of developing the disease in exposed compared to the non-exposed. The risk of exposed individuals may be greater and thus a ratio greater than one would result. There may also be a negative association. This would yield a ratio less than one. A value of one suggests that exposure does not increase risk. Assessing risk either relative or attributable can be a useful endpoint in a study. The presentation of risk as an outcome can be presented as absolute risk. However, often risk outcome is presented as a relative risk reduction which shows a much greater effect than one sees with absolute risk. This may give the impression that the effect is greater than it really is.

Risk can be predicted by a test and be utilized as an outcome measure. We can assess the utility of the test. A useful framework for this assessment is:

	Disease Present	**Disease Absent**
Positive test	true positive	false positive
Negative test	false negative	true negative

One then can assess the sensitivity and the specificity of the outcome of the test.

$$\text{Sensitivity} = \frac{\text{true positives}}{\text{true positives + false negatives}}$$

Thus, sensitivity is the percent with disease with a positive test.

$$\text{Specificity} = \frac{\text{false positive}}{\text{false positives + true negatives}}$$

Thus, specificity is defined as the percent without disease with a negative test.

From these relationships one can assess the positive as well as negative predictive capacity of a test.

Positive predictive value is the probability of disease being present if the test results are positive:

$$\text{Positive predictive value} = \frac{\text{true positive}}{\text{true positive + false positives}}$$

The negative predictive value is the probability of the disease being absent if the test results are negative.

$$\text{Negative predictive value} = \frac{\text{true negative}}{\text{false negative + true negative}}$$

Many studies employ this analysis to assess the utility of a test for a disease state.

Survival Analysis

A very common endpoint employed is survival. One can look at death – (mortality), event free survival, survival or the rate of fatal events. Mortality can be a difficult endpoint making the study analysis difficult because death precludes the occurrence of other endpoints that the patient may have reached if the patient was alive to experience them. In fact, events may not be independent and if the patient lived a second event may have been the cause of the fatality. Sudden death often precludes the diagnosis of an acute myocardial infarction (MI). The MI might have precipitated the sudden death but the patient expires before the MI is identified. This competing risk may be approached by taking competing outcomes into consideration when defining the hazard function in a proportional hazard model.

One can report death as the case fatality rate, the number of total cases in a specified time frame divided by the total number of cases.

A frequently employed representation of mortality is a Kaplan-Meier presentation. This is a graphic depiction of survival during a defied period of observation. The Kaplan-Meier graph establishes a series of intervals with the mortality averaged over each interval. As an example, the mortality in the first month of the study would be graphed with the mortality on the y axis and time on the x access. Each month thereafter, over a defined period, perhaps a year, mortality would be average for each month. But since all patients not studied at the same time, time to death is determined for each patient from the time they started the study and then averaged over each month. At the end of the study those patients who have not died are censored since they have not reached the designated endpoint. While a Kaplan-Meier representation of mortality is very useful as a visual display of outcome (mortality) the analysis does not permit an evaluation for competing risk.

Biomarkers

A biomarker can be defined as a characteristic that is objectively measured and evaluated as an indication of a normal biologic process, pathologic process or pharmacologic response to an intervention. To call a biomarker a surrogate marker the marker must closely correlate with the outcome being measured. The marker must capture the full effect being observed and the marker must be reliably measurable.

An example of a biomarker can be the plaque burden in coronary artery lumen as determined by ultrasound. The plaque burden can be estimated using ultrasound (IVAS). The carotid intima thickness measurements using carotid artery ultrasonography can also be a useful measure of atherosclerosis, a biomarker for the disease. Ventricular Premature Beat (VPC) frequency can be used as a marker for sudden death risk. Tumor size can be a marker for neoplastic disease, or CD4 lymphocyte count as a marker of effective AIDS therapy. All these markers have been considered as indicators of efficacy, though most have limitations. While PVC frequency indicates risk of sudden death in patients with myocardial damage, reducing PVC frequency with anti-arrhythmic drugs available in the 1980's did not correlate with sudden death reduction, but rather an increase in the risk of sudden death (proarrhythmic toxicity). While in some studies IVIS estimation of plaque burden correlated with mortality, in other studies the reduction in plaque by a drug does not correlate with a reduction in mortality. Zidovudine increase CD-4 cells (increase immune function) however this does not correlate with an improved outcome in AIDS patients. A decrease in tumor size may not correlate with an increased survival time in patients with a malignancy. Thus, many biomarkers fail to predict outcome and thus are not surrogate markers. Many biomarkers are thus not useful surrogates to be employed in a study since improvement in the biomarker does not result in an improved outcome.

Perhaps the most useful biomarker that can serve as a surrogate marker is arterial blood pressure. The FDA accepts BP reduction as a marker of drug efficacy. Studies are undertaken with the measurement of outcome being BP not mortality. The medical community accepts BP as an effective target number to treat, believing a reduction in BP will correlate with reduced mortality. But even with BP there are issues. Too great a reduction in BP may lead to adverse outcomes and the measurement itself may not be invariably reliable. Blood pressure readings may be excessively high in the context of a medical office examination (white coat hypertension), but much lower when measured casually at home. Measurements from continuous ambulatory BP recordings may be a better reflection of risk and a better measurement of response to treatment. This suggests that there are nuances to the use of a surrogate biomarker that must be considered when measuring outcomes.

Study Validity

The validity of a study is the extent to which the study reaches a correct conclusion. The internal validity of a study is the extent to which the results of the study truly reflect the study outcome. The interval validity can be affected by false data, lost data, missing data, problems with outcome measures, non-compliance with the study and mistakes in study analysis. External validity is the extent to which the study results are generalizable to the general population, to populations not studied in the trial.

The study outcome measurements can also be affected by bias. A great deal of effort in designing a study is aimed to reduce or eliminate bias. Bias is a systemic error in a study measurement that leads to a distortion of the study results. One could have a selection bias, which is a systemic error due to the patients chosen for the study. One can have a bias due to patients being lost to follow up, or an endpoint being censored or having a competing endpoint. There can be an information bias due to errors in data collection or the falsification of data. Confounding bias occurs when an outcome is distorted by extraneous factors. Biases can severely distort study outcomes and must be eliminated as best as one can by employing effective study design. Selecting the study population, using randomization, ensuing complete follow up of participants, blinding and developing appropriate endpoints that are independent of confounders are all critical.

If one is evaluating a test, one can assess the results by evaluating the reliability of the test. Reliability can be based on the test's accuracy, the number of correct determinations as compared to an absolute standard. One can determine the precision of a test by determining reproducibility and determining the variance in the results.

Example of Outcome Presentations

Say a trial was undertaken to evaluate the effect of a cholesterol lowering agent on death and the study was carried out for 4.9 years.

52/3293 died on placebo = 1.7%

38/3302 died on intervention = 1.2%

absolute risk reduction 1.7 – 1.2 = 0.5%

risk reduction/year 0.5/4.9 = 0.1%/year

The relative risk reduction would be

$$\frac{38/3302}{52/3293} = 72\%$$

and the percentage change in relative risk would be:

100 – 72% = 28%

One could present the outcome in terms of efficacy as the ratio of the placebo rate – treated rate divided by the placebo rate or

$$\frac{1.7 - 1.2}{1.7} = 30\%$$

A metric often not presented but of considerable use to clinicians is the number needed to treat (NNT).

NNT = 1/untreated response – treated response

1/(1.7 – 1.2) = 1/0.005 = 200

Based on this study, the dose of the agent, and its duration of administration one can conclude that in a similar population to that studied the results can be generalized, such that 200 patients would need to be treated to save one life.

Chapter 5

The Population to Study

One can devise an excellent study hypothesis, choose an insightful study design and faithfully execute the study. But if the study population recruited is not what was specified or if recruited very slowly, the study may fail. The selection of the study population is a critical component of any study and must be carefully considered. Unfortunately, there is often no one clear population to select before the study results are known, making decisions in this area difficult. Still consideration of a number of factors can reduce the risk of a failed study.

The study population can be defined as a subset of the population to be evaluated that meets the inclusion and exclusion criteria of the study. The criteria may be very broad or very selective with each of these approaches having benefits and shortcomings. A heterogenous population usually results from less restrictive inclusion and exclusion criteria and is often more generalizable to the total population. This ensures that the findings of a study will be accepted as appropriate for the population being considered for treatment. If one works for a pharmaceutical company, one often strives for the broadest population for the agent to be prescribed. However, as we will see a very heterogenous population may obscure the agent's effectiveness. The drug may only be effective in a subset of the population. A more homogenous population often results from a more restrictive inclusion and exclusion criteria. A more homogeneous population is more likely to share the same pathophysiology, the same precipitating cause of the disease and perhaps a similar genetic background, all influencing the patient's response both in terms of effectiveness and toxicity. There is usually a considerable tension between choosing a more homogenous or a more heterogenous population. Both approaches may have benefits.

The Population Selection Process:

One of the first considerations is to consider who can benefit from the intervention or treatment. It would be obvious that a drug that's target is to lower cholesterol would not be useful in hypertensive patients with a normal cholesterol. A drug that lowers blood pressure may be worth studying in a heart failure population, since BP lowering often improves heart failure. A drug that augments cardiac contractility may be useful in heart failure patients, but in severe heart failure it may increase oxygen consumption, worsening heart failure, causing arrhythmias, and possibly increasing deaths. However, it may not always be clear which population will benefit a priori

Can one detect an effect in the study population is another important consideration? Change is easier to detect in patients with more severe conditions. However, at times those with the most severe conditions may be too advanced in the disease process to show a benefit from treatment. Those with high BP measurements may show a more decisive change than a population with very mild hypertension. It is important to understand the pathophysiology of a disease to make these types of decisions. The stage of heart failure or cancer may be critical. An earlier stage may afford time to permit the agent to show effectiveness independent of the apparent severity of the initial presentation.

Besides utilizing patients with more extreme measurements in the magnitude of the variables being measured to enhance the effect size one can also increase the ability to make effective measurements with other approaches. One can enrich the population with patients who more frequently manifest a given outcome. If one is studying a drug to reduce runs of non-sustained ventricular tachycardia, patients with several episode a day are better to enroll than patients with infrequent episodes (once in 72 hours of recording time). A patient with angina or epileptic seizures with one episode a month would make evaluation of episode frequently difficult. A frequency of once a week would much improve the ability to assess the therapies effect on seizure frequency.

Another approach to “enrich” a study population is to add additional screening factors for the patient population that increase risk. In a study with a cholesterol lowering agent, the population’s risk for events could be increased by including patients with an elevated C-reactive protein, a marker for inflammation. Inflammation has been shown to increase the risk for cardiac events in patients with an elevated cholesterol. In a study I designed for an agent to treat early onset COVID, we included patients with a diagnosis of COVID by antigen testing within 72 hours who were of African American or Hispanic background and had one added risk factor: heart disease, hypertension, obesity or age over 55 years. Self-identified African Americas and Hispanic patients have a 50% increased risk according to the Center for Disease Control (CDC). Having a concomitant risk factor also substantially increased risk. Thus, the COVID study looks at a treatment in a population with an increased number of events predicted, making the effectiveness of a treatment more likely to be observed and the difference between treated and control patients found to be statistically significant.

One reason an effect can't be detected is the absence of the condition being studied or the patient is in a more severe stage of the disease. This can happen by a misdiagnosis or be the result of deception. In a large multinational study in patients with heart failure with preserved ejection fraction (good left ventricular fraction) no benefit was found with spironolactone, a diuretic with anti-fibrotic properties. This is despite benefit reported with heart failure with reduced ejection fraction patients in a previous study though smaller in size. In subsequent analysis it was reported that patients entered in Eastern Europe and Russia did not have heart failure. Not studying heart failure patients puts the negative results of the study in questionable. This skepticism is supported by the evaluation of the North American results that showed a benefit of spironolactone therapy. Unfortunately, the only way to determine if the explanation for the lack of drug efficacy is due to an inappropriate patient population is to repeat the study. A very major and costly undertaking that probably won't happen in the case of heart failure treatment in patients with preserved ejection fraction with spironolactone.

One must take into consideration competing risk in a study population. Patients who may not complete the study due to disease other than the one in question may be censored and distort the study results. A heart failure study most often excludes patients with cancer or severe renal disease who are expected to succumb to those conditions before they succumb to heart failure. Cancer or renal disease deaths would prevent a heart failure endpoint to be met and thus confound the study outcome.

It is important to include patients that one expects to conform to the study protocol. Working in Chicago with so many patients wintering in Florida or Texas alerts one to the need to determine if winter falls during the study period patient needs to be seen and thus they may not adhere to study follow up. Patients who are erratic, showing a labile mood, or have a history of alcohol or drug abuse are often non-compliant. Patients who you have to strenuously “talk into” participating in a study are more likely to be non-compliant with follow up. Patients who have to travel considerable distances may not be compliant, especially in the winter. When working with volunteers as opposed to patients; compliance may be an even greater problem. Patients often perceive a benefit to treatment of their disease as motivation. The contribution patients feel they are making to advance medical knowledge for their disease may also serve as motivation to complete the study. At times volunteers have this altruistic motivation, but volunteers, especially for pharmaceutical Phase I studies participate often for money. At the first sign of inconvenience or difficulty these volunteers may quit the study. Volunteers to enter a study may also withhold information about drug or alcohol use, allergies, or reactions to therapies in other studies in which they participated. One needs to be especially cautious with the "professional" volunteer.

There are ways to improve study population compliance. Careful instructions with study printouts handed out to participants, electronically sent reminders, a dedicated clinical research associate and/or investigators providing encouragement to patients can increase study compliance. However, the study can still fail. One alternative approach is to initiate a "run in" period in the trial. Patients may be followed for a period of time to stabilize them, evaluate their compliance and the veracity of the initial information about their condition. The run-in may be an open untreated period, or it may be on drug therapy. The run-in can access patient compliance as well as drug tolerability. Patients who can't tolerate the therapy can be excluded prior to entry into the definitive part of the study. This of course biases the study to those who tolerate a short course of treatment, possibly reducing side effects reported later in the study. Thus, it is important to note the side effects reported in the "run in" period and the possibility of a selective population, reporting less side effects than that may be seen in the general population. A "run in" resulting in selectivity including responders can also bias the study outcome. This may be an appropriate approach when the therapy may only be effective in a small percentage of the general population. Selecting a sub-population of responder's results in a reduced generalizability of the study findings. What one needs to determine with this approach is the ability to in identify responders to the intervention so physicians in the future can identify the sub-population to treat. This was shown to be useful with the initial work with Herceptin by Genentech in patients with breast cancer. In a general population of women with breast cancer Herceptin, a HER-2 receptor inhibitor was not found to be useful. However, some of the investigators saw a positive signal in patients whose tumor was estrogen receptor negative. They then found that in HER-2 receptor positive patients the drug Herceptin was effective. In selecting breast cancer patients, HER-2 positive breast cancer patients can be identified using the HER-2 receptor as a biomarker for a therapeutic response. The studies in HER-2 positive receptor patients is not generalizable to the entire population with breast cancer. However, the study provides a marker to identify patients who will benefit from Herceptin treatment.

An important tool to evaluate study generalizability is to keep a study screening registry. Recording the screening of each patient and the reason for their inclusion or exclusion can be very useful in the subsequent study analysis. This is especially true with a study with a surprising outcome or a negative outcome that is being questioned as to its validity. Just the number excluded during recruitment tells a lot about the study's generalizability. A study that screens 10,000 candidates for one hundred patients must be suspect as being of limited generalizability. If almost all or all screened patients are entered into a study, the study population is probably generalizable to the entire study population. If all women or black patients are excluded, the study results may not be generalizable to this subset of the population. The screening process can introduce bias that affect the outcome of a study. Knowing how patients were screened and why patients were excluded can be most informative as to study generalizability.

Where one undertakes the study can be a major factor in whom constitutes the study population. A study undertaken in Scandinavia recruits very different patients than one that is commenced in Chicago, USA. A study in heart failure with angiotensin converting enzyme inhibitor (ACE) would recruit a Caucasian Scandinavian population that would be most responsive to ACE therapy while a study recruiting in Chicago in city hospitals would have a very different population with a large number of African Americans who show a lesser response to ACE inhibitors with more reports of angioedema, a serious side effect.

An important consideration is to exclude patients at increased risk or who are vulnerable. Vulnerability can be due to decreased mental capacity (also a consideration for study non-compliance). Vulnerability can be due to being a prisoner, member of the arm services, or patients receiving free medical care. Studies in prisoners are mostly prohibited in federally funded studies and at federal facilities. In some states studies with prisoners are possible with restrictions. Patients who can't understand the consent should be excluded and in individuals who are indecisive, "pushing" them to take part compromises the informed consent process and also will likely lead to a patient "dropping out" of the study at a later date.

Recruitment

Having excessively strict inclusion and exclusion criteria can impair recruitment. Maintaining patient safety is paramount, but excessive exclusions can make recruitment for a study very difficult. Delays in recruitment can increase costs, but even more of a problem is that recruitment delays can lead to changes in the prevailing treatments in the community that effects the study results. A study planned for two or three years that goes on for 5 or more years can be compromised by different background therapies that may have been introduced. Changes in a disease or changes in medical practice or technical expertise are all factors that can alter study outcome. A study should be prosecuted as rapidly as possible. Since study patient recruitment is a major limiting factor, strategies to enhance recruitment are needed and should be planned at the start of a study. It is important to be realistic and not overstate your recruitment capacity. Better to increase the number of investigators sites than to fall way behind in recruitment. If one is unsure that patients can be recruited it may be a reason to initiate a "pilot study". The use of experienced investigators with proven recruitment abilities is advisable, especially with difficult to recruit patient populations. The community in which you are considering undertaking the study may affect recruitment. Communities with less interest in research and those opposed to research or have lingering distrust for research can be a significant problem. It may be advisable to survey the willingness of people in a community as to their interest, support and willingness to participate in clinical research. It is also useful to investigate if other studies recruiting similar patients are being undertake, thus competing with your study. Advertising is an effective, but at times expensive way to recruit patients. Often advertisements attract a lot of volunteers, but many are not appropriate for the study. Obtaining patients from one's practice, the practice of colleagues, a hospital service, or a health care plan can be helpful. One can offer referral inducements though as is the case for patient monetary inducements, this compensation should not be excessive. Giving talks to colleagues, at hospital conferences, to community groups and local patient advocacy groups can be an effective approach to improve recruitment. One can try to involve "thought leaders" to influence referrals. Most useful is employing support staff to recruit patients as well as for them to give talks to nurses and physician assistants to aid in recruitment. Scanning hospital admission records for a diagnosis and then asking the patient's physicians for permission to approach a patient can also be effective. Social media is a new and promising tool for patient recruitment. General advertisements or the use of social media platforms run by patient advocacy groups for a disease can increase recruitment success. Involvement of "managed care" can be very helpful. This often takes time with prolonged reviews, but if one has the cooperation of a managed care group or health plan, the number of patients that can be recruited can be markedly increased.

One needs to approach recruitment as a continuous process that needs to be planned in advance of opening the study. Plans are needed if recruitment does not keep pace with the rate projected. Sites that are not recruiting patients adequately need to receive help to address the specific issues holding back patient recruitment. If the problem can't be corrected those underperforming or non-performing sites should be dropped. Some investigators expend a considerable effort to be involved in a study, obtain IRB approval and then "look around" for patients. Before being involved in a study review one's files to see if you have patients that would meet study entry criteria. If not, it is better for the investigator, the study sponsor and the principal investigator to put their efforts into other sites where success is possible and more likely to occur. Many multicenter studies today work on an auction model. Once an investigator completes all necessary paperwork, obtains IRB approval and organizes and trains staff, accession of patients can occur from a pool of patients. If organized sites with pre-screened patients have used up most of the patient allocation slots, an investigator may only enroll a couple of patients, or even none before the study is closed. A lot of time and effort can be expended with little return with inadequate financial compensation for one's efforts. Identifying patients for a study in advance is needed for successful recruitment.

Monitoring Recruitment Goals

During a study monitoring the pace of recruitment is important. In a multi-center study, the central management team will be monitoring recruitment and will take actions when recruitment falters. One approach to inadequate site recruitment is to accept that the study will take longer to complete, or one may be forced to stop without attaining its enrollment goals. Not obtaining enrollment goals will reduce the power of the study and the likelihood of a definitive outcome. The study may turn out negative, not because the hypothesis was wrong, but because the number of patients enrolled was insufficient to show a positive outcome statistically. Thus, it is far better to try and increase recruitment numbers. Perhaps one can relax inclusion criteria while trying to avoid a significant change in the study population. One may be forced to extend the time for recruitment in a study. This increases the total duration of the study and its costs. An extreme response to failing to enroll enough patients can be to change study design. This is a last resort, but perhaps better than giving up on the study. An often used approach is to try recycling patients who were screening failures. Perhaps the patient was not stable earlier when evaluated and now has stabilized. Perhaps a change in medications can stabilize a patient. For example, one can reduce the BP with medication, so it is not too extreme for patient entry. One also can withdraw one of the patient's medications with their agreement so now they meet the BP entry range for study inclusion or change the number of medications they are using and thus permit the patient to gain entry into the study. Recycling screening failures is often an effective way to enter an additional number of study patients as the end of the enrollment period approaches. Using a stabilization period or medication withdrawal period to meet study entry criteria are also effective approaches.

Special Populations

When designing a study, a special population may be targeted for recruitment to address the study hypothesis. The study may be aimed at a pediatric therapy evaluation and thus pediatric patients may be the target for recruitment. Other special populations may include women of childbearing potential, pregnant women, mentally challenged patients, psychiatric patients, geriatric patients, or patients in acute life-threatening situations. With each of these populations one may have difficulty with the consenting process since these special populations are afforded special protections. There must be appropriate justification for including one of these groups in a clinical trial. Women of childbearing potential may be placed at high risk by an intervention. The mother or child may be placed at risk by a pharmaceutical therapy. Even approved therapies for the general population may not have been studied in pregnant women and thus potentially offer an increased risk. The consent must address these issues and they need to be carefully reviewed by an IRB. Studies are needed in pregnant women, but a careful analysis of the risk vs. benefit needs to be considered before proceeding with such a project. Pediatric research also raises challenges. Individuals under age 18 can't give legal informed consent, consent must be given by a parent or guardian. The age of legal consent is a state issue and can vary. Both federal law when FDA, NIH or NCI is involved, as well as state law must be followed. Children as young as 7 years old may be asked to assent to the research, as well as obtaining legal consent from a parent or guardian. The age of assent can vary with IRB and state regulations.

Prisoners have been studied as a research population and in the past subject to undue influence by authorities. Currently research participation by prisoners is limited by state and federal law. Federal law C.28CFR512.11(a)3 bans research in prisoners “for medical experimentation, cosmetic research or pharmaceutical testing”. Prisoners in state institutions may consent and participate in clinical research depending on the state regulations. If the FDA is involved in regulatory oversight, protection of vulnerable prisoners comes under the IRB and State jurisdiction.

Research in mentally challenged patients is problematic given the potential inability of this population to be able to give informed consent. This population has also been mistreated in the past and is thus considered vulnerable. IRB’s give careful consideration of this groups for participation in clinical research. Patients with Alzheimer’s exhibit a spectrum of competency as to the ability to give informed consent. Having the patient, as well as their “significant other” or legal medical guardian consent gives added protection for the patient and investigator. Psychiatric patients also have difficulty in providing informed consent. It is challenging to determine if the patient is competent to give consent. If the patient’s condition during the study has changed such that they are no longer competent or if the study medication or its stopping may change the cognitive abilities of the patient this may complicate the consenting process. This changing paradigm needs to be considered by the PI and the IRB when planning the consent form and consenting process.

Geriatric patients may also be a vulnerable population. As one ages, a person's cognitive abilities may decrease, and the patient becomes less able to evaluate the risks and benefits of a study. Elderly patients are known to be far more susceptible to "confidence scams" and can be unduly influenced. Also, elderly patients are more frail and thus subject to a greater number of adverse side-effects from experimental treatments. For these reasons the feasibility of studies in the elderly needs to be evaluated in terms of the risk to the participant and the participant's ability to give informed consent.

Another vulnerable population are patients in extremes, patients undergoing a medical emergency, or patients who are not mentally alert due to neurologic injury. In the chapter on the IRB we will discuss how to study these patients without obtaining consent. Certainly, studies are much needed in this patient population. There have been recent changes in the legal procedure for research when a patient is having an emergency. It is possible in this type of research to waive the consenting process. Undertaking studies that bypass the consent process is a complicated undertaking involving community notification, appropriate justification, IRB and FDA approval (if a drug or device study is involved) and the NIH if it is providing grant support for the study.

Participation of a non-study affiliated physician assessing that the patients meet the criteria for study entry is also needed.

Research in special populations despite being more complex is certainly needed. Research needs to include women, patients with impaired hepatic and renal function, and patients on multiple drugs (polypharmacy). Failing to study these patients makes a therapeutic evaluation problematic with reduced generalizability.

Chapter 6. The Study Protocol and Investigator Brochure

A clinical trial requires a protocol that provides the necessary information to undertake the trial. A person new to the study should be able to understand the reason for the trial, its objective and how to carry out the study. A protocol is not meant to teach a novice how to practice medicine, preform a cardiac catheterization, or read an EKG. Investigators qualified to undertake the study must have the necessary knowledge and skills required to carry out the study. However, the study procedures need to be clearly and completely explained in the study protocol. Some large, multi-center studies have a manual to accompany a protocol that describes aspects of the highly technical aspects of the study such as packaging a lab's samples for shipment to a central laboratory or specifications and calibration for diagnostic equipment to be used in the study. Most studies don't need this degree of detailed information.

Hypothesis

A statement of the primary hypothesis that is clear and amenable to testing should be initially stated followed by an enumeration of secondary hypothesis that are pre-specified.

Background of the Study

A clear and concise description of the reason for understanding the study and its significance should be included in the background section. What studies have been performed to-date and how do they differ from the current study. What were the problems with earlier studies and how does the current study provide additional information? A description of the state of medical care for the condition being studied, where the study will be performed and required background therapies. Explaining the design of the study and why some therapies are given to all patients and some not is important to discuss.

Table 1. The Study Protocol

I Hypothesis
- a) Primary question
- b) Secondary question(s)

II Background of the Study
- a) Significance of question
- b) Previous studies on this or related topics
- c) Problems with earlier studies
- d) Reason to undertake study

III Study Design
- a) What type of study is it
- b) Blinded
- c) Control
- d) Study population
- e) Duration of study
- f) Randomization

IV Entry into Study

a) Inclusion criteria

b) Exclusion criteria

V Study Procedures

a) Baseline

b) Schedule of treatments

c) Schedule of procedures

d) Study visit schedule

e) Site training

f) Monitoring schedule

VI Data Collection

a) Who collects data

b) When does it take place

c) Data forms (electronic or paper)

d) Quality control procedures

e) Adverse event reporting

VII Study Stopping and Termination

a) When does study end

b) Early termination – reasons, who can terminate study

c) What are the termination procedures and how implemented

VIII Administration

a) PI and role

b) Sub-investigator(s) role

c) Is there a data safety monitoring committee

d) Sponsor role and funding

IX Informed Consent & HIPA Form

X References

XI Appendices

a) Core labs

b) Study definitions

c) Emergency procedures, contacts

d) Data collection forms

e) Internet security procedures

f) Randomization system directions

Study Design

What type of study is the one being undertaken, parallel vs. crossover for example? Is the study randomized, does the study have a control arm? Is the study blinded? What population is being evaluated and for how long are patients to be followed? What randomization system is employed? Is the randomization 1 to 1 ratio or 2 to 1 (intervention vs. control), or some other allocation ratio employed?

Entry into Study

A statement of the inclusion and exclusion criteria employed in the study. The criteria for inclusion or exclusion should be stated as clearly as possible to avoid potential violations.

Study Procedures

Describe what will be done and in what order. A table or flow chart is most useful. Anyone carrying out the study should be able from the study procedures understand what needs to be done and the next step for each patient in the study. What are the baseline procedures, when is consent obtained, when does randomization occur, when does the patient receive treatment, what dose of medication is used to initiate therapy? What happens if patient misses a treatment or a dose of the study medication? When are study visits to be scheduled and make up visits scheduled if a study visit is missed (which can frequently happen, especially in cold and snowy Chicago winters)? Who trains the study personnel? When and how are study procedures updated or changed as in study amendments? What is the monitoring schedule of the study and what is expected at each monitoring session? Who needs to be present at each visit and who needs to be available if the study is to be monitored by a central body or external group (company, DSMB, FDA or NIH?)?

Data Collection

How is the data collected, who undertakes the data collection? Is data collected in person? Are electronic data system employed?

How is adverse event reporting done? What are the responsibilities as to serious adverse event reporting; to sponsor, central management committee, local or central IRB? How is quality of data insured. Who monitors and what quality control procedures are incorporated in the study?

Study Pausing or Termination

Why would the study be terminated? Who can terminate the study? Who can stop or pause the study, for what reasons and when and can the study can be re-started once paused and who determines restarting? There can be a very simple, straightforward rules for a single site study or a complex set of rules for a multi-center study with a Data Safety Monitoring Committee, an Executive Committee, a PI, an Administrative Group, and a Congress of Investigators. There needs to be stated responsibilities, designated authorities and mechanisms of appeal in the protocol with these more complicated studies.

Study Administration

Who is the Principal Investigator (PI), what is the PI's role and in multi-center studies how is the PI chosen? Who are the sub-investigators, what are their roles in the study? How can a site and/or its principal investigator be terminated? Who can order a site closed and is there an appeal process? Is there a Data Safety Monitoring Committee and what are its responsibilities and powers? Most multi-center studies have a DSMB, studies under FDA and NIH purview are mostly required to have a DSMB. IRB's are requiring a Data Safety Monitoring Plan that often may include a DSMB or forming one depending on an independent interim analysis of the study. What are the procedures for activating a DSMB?

It is appropriate to describe the source of funding for the study: NIH, NCI, academic institution, pharmaceutical industry, device company, or a private sponsor. The source of funding should be stated, as well as if the sponsor is in charge of the study. Is the sponsor involved in running the day-to-day activities of the study or is the study independent of the sponsor?

Informed Consent and the HIPPA Form

A copy of the informed consent should be attached to the protocol. There is usually an informed consent model that is provided to sites to draft into their local IRB's format. When submitting a study protocol as part of an IND submission there is often a consent included that has not been reviewed or approved by an IRB. Multi-center studies may often employ a central IRB and once approval of the study protocol occurs with an approved consent, these documents can be incorporated in the protocol along with changes in the protocol mandated by the IRB. A multi-center study employing multiple IRB's may not include the multiple different versions of consents that may have minor differences. However, substantial changes in the protocol, and those with changes involving the inclusion and exclusion of patients need to be harmonized before the study can commence.

As of 1996 each patient needs to be provided with a Health Insurance and Portability and Accountability Act (HIPA) form to review and sign. The document informs the patient of their rights regarding their protected health information and how can the protected health information be used by the investigators.

The HIPA form is a legal document and can limit the access of information to those administering the study. The HIPA form needs to be carefully written to give access to the patients protected health information and databases with patient information even if the patient withdraws from the study. This information can include hospital records and death certificate information, so patient outcome can be reported in a study. The Office of Protection of Human Research (OPHR) that oversees human research permits the Consent and HIPPA forms to be combined. I believe that this is easier for the patient than being explained the reasons for two separate documents and having to read both.

References and Appendix

A protocol is not a scholarly publication and for this reason hundreds of references are not required. One should reference those statements that are controversial or where a reference paper will provide additional study background for those interested. A reference to a complex or new technique can be helpful to the participating physicians to gain additional information. The appendices can be used for multiple purposes. One can insert flow sheets, data collection forms, core lab information, methods of study specimen storage, information on shipment to a central lab, methods used in an electronic data form, internet security procedures and emergency procedures and contacts. Forms for adverse events (AE) and serious adverse events (SAE) reporting can be included. Many studies have complex definitions, and the appendix is a place to list these operational definitions. As an example, the protocol may require the diagnosis of an acute MI. The appendix is the place to define the ECG charges required, the type of troponin test and threshold for MI diagnosis and the laboratory result threshold needed to state the patient is positive for an MI. It should be stated if blood samples are to be saved, sent to a central site for storage or disposed of at the study site.

The Study Brochure

Most study protocols involving pharmaceuticals or devices are required to have an accompanying Investigator's Brochure. Many IRB's require an Investigator's Brochure if a therapy or device is being studied even if the device or drug has been approved. This is especially the case if an approved drug or device is being studied for an off-label use.

Table II. The Investigator's Brochure (IB) for Pharmaceuticals

I) Introduction
   a) Background
   b) Reason for investigation

II) Properties of the Drug
   a) Physical properties
   b) Chemical properties
   c) Formulation

III) Pre-Clinical Studies

a) Pharmacology

b) Kinetics

c) Metabolism

d) Toxicology

IV) Studies in Man

a) Kinetics

b) Metabolism

c) Efficacy studies

d) Safety reports

e) Planned studies

V) Outside U.S. study results and approvals

VI) Regulatory status

VII) Publications

VIII) Reverences

The Study Brochure

Introduction

The Investigator's Brochure starts with a discussion of the field being studied, the background information of the area being investigated, the therapeutic entity and how it differs from current therapy. The reason for initiating the investigation and the intended goals (development of a new drug or new indication of an approved drug).

Properties of the Drug

The basic properties of the drug should be described. Its physical, chemical properties of the compound as well as the other compounds in the formulation (diluents, stabilizers).

Pre-Clinical Studies

A description of pre-clinical studies should be presented, especially those studies required for human investigation. Basic pharmacology studies along with studies that characterize the drug's pharmacokinetics that justify the current dosing strategy to be employed in the study. The metabolites of the drug, metabolic byproducts and if known active metabolites. The pathway (renal, hepatic) of clearance should be described. Animal toxicology and teratogenicity studies should be summarized. A summary for each area is sufficient for the IB.

Studies in Man

What studies have been done in man, at what dose and for how long should be stated. A brief description of the study and its results should be provided. What side effects were encountered and in what frequency. Studies that are "first in man" followed by kinetic studies and then efficacy studies should be reported. Findings as to human absorption, distribution, metabolism and elimination should be reported. Were there any serious adverse reactions reported, especially death or hospitalization. What studies are planned and why should be discussed.

Outside the U.S. Studies

Is the drug approved or being studied outside the U.S. and if so, what studies, what efficacy and safety findings have been reported in OUS studies?

Regulatory Studies

Are studies planned to fulfil regulatory requirements or are they completed and if so, the studies should be described. What IND studies are planned (Phase I, II, III). Was NDA submitted. Are additional Phase IV studies planned or being undertaken? Is an approved drug being studied for a new indication and thus the subject of a second IND filing? Is this study part of a supplemental NDA?

Publications:

A list of all publications with the drug to-date should be provided.

References:

Citations in IB should be listed in the reference section.

Table III. Investigator's Brochure for Devices

- I) Introduction
  - a) Background
  - b) Reasons for study(s)
- II) Properties of Device
  - a) Overview of engineering
  - b) Number of iterations of device thus far

c) Description of software employed

d) Protection of device from hacking or unauthorized interrogation

III) Pre-clinical In Vitro studies

a) Summary of In Vitro testing

b) Safety studies

IV) Studies in Man

a) First in man testing

b) Efficacy studies

c) Safety studies

d) Planned studies for approval

V) Studies outside U.S.

a) Efficacy

b) Safety

c) What countries is the device approved or pending approval

VI) Regulatory studies

a) In progress

b) Undertaken

VII) Software Considerations

a) Summary of development

b) Alpha testing results

c) Beta testing results

d) Security of software

VIII) Publications

IX) References

The Device Brochure is similar to an IB for drugs with pertinent sections on emergency procedures, in vitro testing, performance standards and consideration of software updates with security protections related to the devices software. While a drug can't be modified once an IND is submitted (a new agent would start the process all over) a devise goes through many iterations and a description of each and the reasons for these changes should be in the IB. Given the regulatory procedures in the EU, most devices receive a quick C-mark in Europe and thus a lot of data is accumulated in Europe before U.S. studies commence. For this reason, the outside the U.S. (OUS) Studies in Man section should be as complete as possible to inform U.S. investigators of prior experience with the device and what iteration was used in each study and what side effects if any were observed.

A description of previous adverse events associated with the device should be included in the IB.

Chapter 7.
Sample Size and the Power Calculation

How one measures endpoints will determine the method of calculating a sample size – the numbers to be studied in order to have a statistically reasonable chance of a successful study outcome. Data endpoints may be categorical, continuous, or a rate to an endpoint. A successful study is one that rejects the null hypothesis and accepts the alternative hypothesis. A credible chance of success is having an 80% ability (power) to find a significant difference at the $p<0.05$ level. The most frequently employed technique for data analysis is based on the premise that statistical inference can be drawn from data by determining the frequency of the occurrence(s). This is called the frequentist approach. An alternative approach is called Bayesian where probabilities of events can be estimated by data collected as a study progresses based on previous probabilities (posterior probability). A frequentist approach would have an assumption about the frequencies or distribution of collected data, project the sample size and then when the data is collected following the protocol having been analyzed, the data will be evaluated employing established statistical techniques. The tests are based on the characteristics of the data; continuous or categorical and the number of comparisons made. The Bayesian approach would be to take what is known, make sample size assumptions based on prior experience and then as the study progresses make sample size adjustments to take into account the new information obtained.

There was a time where most clinical studies were done following a frequentists approach. While the majority of studies are still performed using a frequentist statistical approach, Bayesian approaches are being utilized much more frequently. The Bayesian approach permits adjustments to changing circumstances and may be especially helpful in studies where information to base effect size estimates is limited or lacking. However, a Bayesian approach can be considerably more complex to carry out with the need for greater statistical knowledge and usually professional statistical help.

Why try to estimate sample size

For a study to be impactful one needs to be able to say the findings did not occur by chance and that the study had the ability (power) to assess a statistically successful outcome. Without an adequate sample size to yield a statistically significant outcome one leaves the study success to chance. Many studies are underpowered and can't resolve the study hypothesis. Why undertake such a study since you are putting resources, your time and effort into a project that is unlikely to be successful. More important is that you are asking patients to take part in a study with a low probability of answering the study hypothesis, but still asking the patients to assume the risks the study might pose. An underpowered study for this reason may be unethical as well as futile. When we use established parameters of an 80% power, we are still accepting a 20% chance of being underpowered to reach a definitive conclusion. Accepting the 0.05 or less alpha level assumes a false positive result could occur by chance in 1 out of 20 instances. This possibility of making a mistake is quite liberal indeed. To go for more power and an increased statistical chance of not having a false positive is going to require a much larger sample size that may not be feasible. Sample size determination is a compromise between the feasible and the risk of a false positive.

The Sample Size

To determine sample size, one needs to base the sample on a response variable in the study. This is the primary response variable that is central to the study hypothesis. The response variable can be continuous, dichotomous, or time to an outcome. When one conceptualizes a study, one determines the kind of response variable to obtain and then choose an appropriate test to determine if the difference between the treated group and the untreated group are different and if their difference is statistically significant. When we are evaluating the sample size, we don't know the actual data that is to be obtained, but we do know our assumptions for power and statistical validity, the p value we will accept. Using these parameters and an estimate of the effect size we can employ the formula for obtaining statistical significance and calculate for the sample size (n). What is critical in a sample size evaluation is the estimation of effect size. This is not a guess or an enthusiastic estimate, but a conservative assessment based on prior experience. Perhaps there is a similar study performed or a similar population studied for a similar outcome giving an understanding of the potential outcome, its variability and its effect size. The variability (standard deviation) is very important in assessing sample size since the effect size relates to the number needed to study modified by the variability around the point estimate. The more variability encountered the larger the sample size.

Investigators are often enthusiastic with the chosen treatment and have overly optimistic effect size estimates. Experienced investigators often say that an effect size greater than 20% is unrealistic. Additionally, a variance around the effect size in rarely less than 10%, and may often be 20%, or even up to 50%. Imprecise measurements of the outcome variable, increased missing data, patients “dropping out” or lost to follow up may all combine to increase variability. The inherent differences in biology of patients in the studies may contribute to variability, necessitating a larger sample size. Assessing the point estimate and variability in terms of available data from similar studies, studies in similar populations and studies employing the same or similar measurement tools is essential to an appropriate estimation of sample size.

Dichotomous Variables

Dichotomous variables can be independent of each other, or they can be paired. Most dichotomous variables are independent.

One takes the statistical test equation, in this case for a dichotomous variable and solves the equation for N.

$$Z = (Pc - Pi) / \sqrt{\overline{P}(1 - \overline{P})\,(1/Nc + 1/Ni)}$$

Pi = event rate in intervention

Pc = event rate in control

N = number of participants (N_c – control, N_i – intervention)

$\overline{P} = (Pc + Pi) / 2$

Z is comprised of two components ($Z\alpha$ and $Z\beta$)

$Z\,\alpha$ = critical value that corresponds to the significance level of α

$Z\,\beta$ = value not exceeded by probability β

$$2\,N = 4(Z\alpha + Z\beta)^2\,\bar{p}\,(1 - \bar{p}) / (p_c - p_i)^2$$

Table I Value of $Z\alpha$

α	one sided	2-sided test
0.05	1.645	1.960
0.01	2.326	2.576

Value of $Z\beta$

Power	$Z\beta$
80%	0.84
90%	1.282
95%	1.645

Example: Comparing an outcome (perhaps an MI) in the control group (Pc) with that in the intervention group (Pi).

Pi = 30%= 0.30 Pc =40%=0.4

2 sided test $\alpha = 0.05$

80% power

$Z\alpha = 1.96$

$Z\beta = 0.84$

$\bar{p}$= (0.30+0.40)/2 = 0.35

Using the equation above ($2N = 4(Z\alpha + Z\beta)^2\, \bar{p}\,(1 - \bar{p}) / (p_c - p_i)^2$)

$2N = 4(1.96+0.84)^2 0.35(1-0.35)/(0.4-0.3)^2 \approx 714$

N= 357 patients in each group

Sample size calculation for continuous variable

$$Z = (\bar{X}c - \bar{X}i) / \sigma \sqrt{1/NC + 1/Ni}$$

$$2N = 4(Z\alpha + Z\beta)^2\, \sigma^2 / \delta^2$$

Nc = number control

Ni = number intervention

σ = variance

δ = expected change (effect size)

Example: A study evaluating a change in BP between control and intervention.

10 mmHg BP change $\alpha = 0.05$

15 mmHg variance power = 80%, $Z_\beta = 0.84$

$2N = 4(1.96 + 0.84)^2 (15)^2 / (10)^2$

$2N = 70$

$N = 35$ patients in each group

If one wants to adjust for patients who "drop out" and for patients who change form control to intervention group ("drop in's").

$N_c = N/(1 \text{ --}Ro - Ri)^2$

Ro = dropouts R_i – drop in's

Example: If Ro = 10 % = 0.1 and R_i =5%= 0.05

$35/ (1-0.1- 0.05)^2$ = adjusted sample size = 48 patients in each group required with a power of 80%.

Sample size for time to event (survival analysis)

λ hazard rate

λc = control rate

λi = intervention rate

$$2N = \frac{4(Z\alpha + Z\beta)^2}{\ln(\lambda c/ \lambda_i)^2}$$

Example: In a study the morbidity is 15% (control rate) and the rate in the intervention rate is 10%

$4(Z\alpha - Z\beta)^2 = 4(1.96+0.84)^2 = 31.4$

$\lambda c / \lambda_i = 0.15 / 0.1 = 1.5$

$(\lambda c / \lambda_i)^2 = 1.5^2 = 2.25$

$\ln 2.25 = 0.81$

$2N = 31.4/0.81 = 38.7 \approx 39$

Considering two equal groups of patients, 20 patients will be enrolled into each group, for a total of 40 patients.

Practical Alternative Approaches

Most researchers utilize sample size calculators. These are easy to find with a simple search on the internet. Some examples are listed below.

Dichotomous variables:

- sample_size.net
- clincalc.com
- sphweb.bumc.bu.edu

Continuous variables:

- pharmaschool.com
- sealedenvelope.com
- statpowers.com

Hazard ratio:

gigacalculator.com

sample-size.net

powerandsamplesize.com

Estimation Difficulties

The estimates needed to perform sample size calculations can be difficult and very perplexing to develop when prior studies are not available. But this is often the case when a new, novel study is planned. There may be small studies reported in the literature, but by virtue of their size, the point estimate and variance may be considerably off. It is also important to know that the outcome measurements (death, hospitalization, etc) as regards disease frequency are reduced in randomized clinical trials probably because of the exclusion criteria employed (overly protective) and partly because of greater comprehensive care provided in the clinical trial setting. Thus, by extrapolating from an observational study to a randomized controlled trial the process is fraught with difficulty and may lead to underestimation of the required sample size. Another consideration in the sample size calculation is that it can be based on small differences that may be significant but are not clinically meaningful. One does not want to initiate a study and find the results significant but not clinically meaningful.

One approach to increasing the accuracy of the sample size estimation is to undertake a pilot study. The results of the pilot would not be definitive, but the estimation of effect size and its variability would greatly increase the accuracy of a sample size calculation for the definitive trial. A pilot study also supports the feasibility of carrying out the study and may lead to modifications in study procedures and measurement metrics used to determine outcome. Pilot studies take time and are costly, so they are usually employed in novel areas with sizable financial support available to the investigator. A pilot study can be an external pilot where the study is separate and distinct from the proposed larger study and is undertaken primarily as a feasibility study. An internal pilot can also be undertaken to determine feasibility and provides data for sample size estimation. However, the initial pilot is performed in an identical manner as to the proposed larger study and the internal pilot's data is planned to be combined with the larger study data for a combined analysis. This approach conserves resources, reduces overall costs and may reduce the time to obtain the outcome results.

Chapter 8

Blindness and Randomization

A clinical trial takes a considerable investment of time, effort and money as well as asking people to participate when they are often faced with difficult circumstances due to their medical condition. Everything needs to be done to see that a clinical study reaches a correct conclusion. Biases can cause a study to fail, not reaching a correct conclusion and thus every effort needs to be made to prevent biases from undermining a study. Two actions an investigator can take to minimize bias is to blind the study and use effective randomization techniques.

Blindness

Blinding is a technique that can greatly reduce the problem of bias, the systematic introduction of error into a study. All studies have an inherent variability. However, this variability can be exaggerated by bias that can lead to a false negative result or a false positive outcome. By removing the knowledge of the intervention, the patient's and the investigator's influence on the outcome of the study can be greatly reduced.

A study can be unblinded and thus the patient as well as the investigator know the intervention that the patient is receiving. The patient may be influenced by the knowledge that they are receiving the active treatment. It is not just psychological outcomes that can be distorted by knowledge of the intervention, but physiologic conditions. Blood pressure can be influenced by knowing the treatment. Anginal frequency can be affected by knowledge that the patient is receiving active therapy. Patients undergoing an operation are more likely to believe the intervention offers benefit. As an example, the Vineberg procedure of anastomosing an artery to the myocardium was reported to relieve otherwise untreatable angina through there is no blood flow to the ischemic myocardium. The mind does wonders!

A single blind study is one where the patient is unaware of the intervention, but the investigators are knowledgeable. This reduces the biases that the patient can introduce to change outcome, but it does nothing to limit the biases of the investigators. An investigator may feel a patient is too sick to receive a placebo or a perceived inferior standard therapy and thus bias the study by putting healthier patients into the control group. Conversely an investigator may feel the need to only place healthier patients into the intervention group and thus bias the study possibly favoring the control group. Or the bias may be a more subtle one where the investigator feels bad that the control group fails to receive the "better" intervention, the new treatment being studied and thus gives the control group more rigorous care, once again biasing the study. Any way you look at a single blind study the potential for bias makes this a poor choice.

A double-blind trial is one where neither the patient nor the investigator or the investigational staff knows the allocation of the patient to active treatment being studied or control. This prevents the patient or the investigator to easily introduce their biases that may influence study outcomes. This is certainly the preferred study design. While some argue that the physician needs to know the intervention or drug being studied to protect the patient. This is not true. Knowing the treatment or drug is no substitute for careful patient monitoring and exercising good medical judgement. It is easy to assume potential outcomes as result of therapy being both good and bad, that in reality have no relation to the actual outcome. Knowing the therapy just introduces biases, both in favor and against the intervention. Better to practice medicine and be a careful observer than a biased activist. With the frequent use of the double-blind study design and the frequent undertaking of large multi-centered trials the need for a data monitoring plan has become mandatory by IRB's and the utilization of a Data Monitoring Safety Board (DSMB), to be discussed in detail in a subsequent chapter. The DSMB is looked upon as substituting for the blinded researcher in surveilling the study and insuring patient safety.

A triple-blind study is one where neither the patient, the investigator, or the DSMB knows which intervention the patient is receiving. This is the strictest study design to prevent bias. The bias of the patient, the investigators, and the members of the DSMB are blocked from biasing the study. A triple-blind study ensures that the study outcome is unlikely to be due to the introduction of bias. Many argue that a triple-blind study is unethical because the DSMB that serves as a surrogate for the investigator in ensuring patient safety is blinded and can't function effectively. This is just nonsense. If you believe a double-blind study is necessary to remove investigator bias, then a triple-blind study is needed to prevent the introduction of biases from the DSMB. Substituting the DSMB biases for the investigator biases makes no sense. So, then who is "looking out" for the patients? The answer is that both the investigators and the DSMB. The investigator sees the patients frequently and are the first in line to intervene and if needed to stop a study and report adversity to the IRB, study sponsor and if applicable FDA or NIH. They react much faster to serious adversity since they are directly on scene while a DSMB meets 2 or 3 times a year at most and takes months to receive and evaluate the ongoing study data. Even urgently convening a DSMB meeting adds considerable delay. However, the DSMB does have a better picture of overall study trends, both in terms of efficacy and safety. It is the DSMB's responsibility to issuing warnings, more intense monitoring and patient surveillance guidelines or if needed to stop the study. Knowing which treatment the patient is receiving can only bias the DSMB. The guidelines should be arbitrary not dependent on treatment knowledge. Too many studies have been stopped due to DSMB biases leaving the medical field littered with incomplete answers to critical medical questions.

An example of how a major trial that greatly influenced cardiology can be looked at in terms of DSMB blinding is the CAST trial. Before this trial VPC's were a known marker for risk for sudden death and it was widely believed that suppressing VPC's with the then available or in development anti-arrhythmics would reduce mortality. Early in the study an adverse trend was noted. Investigators did not know the treatment arm the adverse trend in mortality was occurring since the study was double-blind. However, the DSMB was not blinded and stopped one arm and then the entire study. Did the DSMB need to know what therapy the adverse mortality trend was occurring? Once the pre-set boundary for adversity was crossed, the study should be terminated. If it turned out that the adverse mortality was in the control arm of the study, then the interventions would be considered effective and it being unethical to continue the study since not treating patients for their VPC's would be unethical. It turned out that the mortality was higher in the group receiving anti-arrhythmic therapy, undercutting the hypothesis that treatment of VPC's with anti-arrhythmics would reduce the incidence of sudden death. The boundary that was pre-set was crossed and the study needed to be stopped. A trial with the DSMB knowing the outcome could early on trend in the wrong direction leading to a premature termination, leaving an unanswered question. Are we demanding that patients be kept in studies with potential harm to obtain definitive answers to important medical questions? The answer is a resounding **NO**. We are just asking for appropriate, reasonable boundaries to be pre-established that reduce the chance of biases or a trend occurring by chance in an adverse direction causing the study to be terminated. It may be with the results may turn in favor of the investigational therapy. Trends in the outcome often change and knowing the treatment assignments tends to arouse irresistible behavior and impassioned pleas to intervein by stopping the study.

It should be pointed out that in most outcome studies the control arm(s) is not usually a placebo but "standard of care", established therapy, and thus keeping patients receiving control arm therapy for a prolonged period does not pose an inordinate risk. Being on the intervention could in fact introduce harm and that is why a boundary is established such that if crossed terminates the study.

Assessment of Blindness

An assessment of the effectiveness of the study design by the evaluation of the blinding techniques is often overlooked. It is de regur to say the study is blinded but was it really blinded. Patient's may know if they are receiving active drug. The investigator may have inadvertently broken the blind through clues in lab tests, or perhaps actively broken the blind during the study. It is useful to evaluate if the blind has been maintained by asking the patients and the investigators which group the patients were in during the study. In a large trial this can be done by sampling patients from the various centers. Breaking the blind may be inadvertent due to a number of factors such as the taste of the placebo pill. If a study blind has been broken, partially or completely it does not invalidate the study but should be known and taken into consideration in interpreting the study results.

Study Randomization

Randomization of a study plays an important part in limiting bias as well as helping ensure that the study groups are comparable in known and unknown factors that can influence study outcome. Randomization when implemented effectively removes investigator bias as well as participant bias. The standard tests a "frequentist" uses is based upon the assumption that the groups in the study are formed by random assignment. There are two major forms of bias. Selection bias is when the allocation to study group assignment is not random. Non-random allocation permits a selection bias to enter into the study. Randomization and blindness prevent the introduction of selection bias since which group receives the intervention is not known (blindness) and the allocation is by chance. A second form of bias is accidental bias. Randomization does not always allocate participants in a study in a balanced way. Known or unknown characteristics of a patient that can influence outcome may not be evenly distributed in the allocation process. The larger the study the more likely the allocation is evenly distributed. Studies of 10, 25, 50 patients are not likely to evenly distribute patients with different characteristics. Studies of 100 or more patients is more likely but this is not always the case, especially when there are multiple factors influencing outcome. In a heart failure trial, the degree of heart failure (class II, III or IV) greatly effects outcome regardless of therapy. If patients are not distributed equally between groups, the state of the patient's heart failure may determine outcome over that of the effect of treatment. Thus, techniques to ensure an equal distribution of critical factors is essential to ensure an unbiased outcome. To achieve a random distribution there are a number of available techniques.

Types of Randomizations

Randomization means allocation by chance, the process not being predictable. The simplest way to achieve randomization is to flip a coin each time, for a study with two groups, heads means one group and tails the other. After a few flips of the coin there will be an imbalance, but this imbalance will disappear after hundreds of coin flips. But there can still be an imbalance due to involvement of multiple centers in recruitment or recruitment under different conditions at different times. Say the centers are involved in a heart failure trial. One center is run by a leading heart failure cardiologist who is referred the “sickest of the sick” and second site is a teaching hospital that infrequently undertakes research, and the third site is a busy community cardiology practice. The “maven” site has the patients all lined up, enters a large number of the sickest patients early on with an initial imbalance between the 2 groups. The research teaching hospital that is less primed for the process takes 6 months to obtain IRB approval and enters only few patients mostly severely ill as well. The community practice comes in late but has a large volume of patients with mild disease. Even those severe patients (Class IV) are much less ill than the “maven” site Class IV heart failure patients. The site with less ill patients may not be able to correct the imbalance that may have occurred early on resulting from the first site and thus one of the study arms may end up with sicker patients than the other which can greatly affect outcome. There are straightforward randomization approaches that can prevent such a situation from developing.

Fixed Allocations

In a two-arm study one can have an equal allocation between the two groups or an unequal one. The choice depends upon the aim of the study and the investigators additional objectives. If the study is to establish efficacy say of a new drug, then an equal allocation is preferred. If the goal is to establish efficacy and observe the effects of long-term treatment, then it makes sense to place more patients in the active therapy group. If the blind is maintained, then there is no loss of equipoise. If there are more than two groups, one can have equal or unequal allocation among groups. The critical consideration is that unequal allocations occur with the blind maintained. This can be done with the treatment medication **not** known and the number in each group blinded to the investigators. If there is any identifier for one therapy over the other to help distinguish therapy, then if it is known the active therapy is administered twice as often as control then the blind can easily be broken. The frequency of one therapy over another needs to be concealed and the therapies indistinguishable.

Simple Randomization:

One approach to randomization is to allocate each patient one at a time to one of the groups. This can be done by flipping a coin, using a random number table or a computer program that generates a random allocation. With small numbers in each group (less than 50) one can develop allocation imbalances up to 20%. Thus, simple allocation is not an advisable method when one is studying small numbers of patients. If one wants to employ this method, one can use Microsoft Excel random number calculator or turn to an "on line" system. https://www.random.org/lists/ .

To prevent an allocation imbalance one can, employ the technique of block randomization. One randomizes in "blocks" of a selected length such that the order of the block is selected on a random basis. The number of allocations in each block divided by 2 is the maximum imbalance that can exist using this technique. This method is especially useful if a study is stopped abruptly. The imbalance will not be greater than the block size, number of random allocations divided by 2. An example would be a block size of eight (ABBBABAA), A being one group and B being the other. The imbalance of allocations to group A or B can never be greater than 4 allocations. All the allocations (blocks) are created on a random basis. One can turn to an "on-line calculator" to undertake block randomization. https://www.sealedenvelope.com/simple-randomiser/V1/list or, alternatively a "block randomization generator":
http://www.jerrydallal.comrandom/random_block_sice_r.htm

This site also has a random sequence generator that can be useful when you want to randomize to two treatments but also want to randomize the treatment sequence such as doses in a bioequivalence trial. In such a trial the first patient receives treatment A and for a repeat treatment would receive treatment B. Then one would randomize the next patient randomly to the alternative treatment with the order of the sequence randomized as well (IV vs. oral or generic drug vs. innovator).

Stratified Randomization

There may be significant patient factors that can influence outcome. Thus, randomly allocating patients to one or the other treatment group may not create a balance among those factors. One group may have more patients with attributes that affect outcome in one direction and thus biases the study. One can correct for this potential imbalance if one knows the factors that are important to establish balance between the two groups. The process of taking these factors into consideration is called stratification. This can be done in the randomization process or in the analysis phase after the study is complete. The advantage of doing the balancing in advance is the ability to control sub-group size. After the study is over one can't increase the size of a stratified group. One can decide to increase the study size if one finds that the stratified groups are too small to analyze with meaningful statistical certainty. In a heart failure study, heart failure class and the presence of diabetes (Type II) greatly affect outcome and thus you want the treatment group and the control group to be balanced for these factors. You may decide that you need 25 patients in each stratum (3 heart failure groups) each with or without diabetes or a total of 6 strata. You can adjust the size of the study to account for these factors and you can randomize patients into the 6 strata on a random basis permitting an unbiased assessment of the intervention vs placebo in mild, moderate, and severe heart failure with or without Type II diabetes. If one does not know the factors that can affect outcome and only learns of these issues after the study, one can perform a stratified analysis.

Adaptive Randomization Techniques

Adaptive techniques adjust the randomization process on the basis of the prior randomization results; thus the process is adaptive. These techniques are less utilized because they are more difficult to carry out and may have some unwanted consequences.

One technique often called the "biased coin" technique is an attempt to adjust the next randomization allocation based on the prior randomization. As the probability of randomization differs 50/50 from a randomization based on the prior randomization results one increases the odds of one group over the other, to adjust the probability closer to 50/50 balance. One can adjust the probability slowly over the course of the study or the adjustment can be completed on the next patient randomization.

A second approach is called the "Urn Design" which adjusts the probability in real time. Imagine an "urn" with equal number of A and B balls representing allocations of patients in a study. As you pick one, say A and allocate to one study arm then one increases the possible next allocation by returning the A ball to the urn and add an additional B ball, increasing the probability of selecting a B just a bit. One can add a stratification process to this adaptive randomization though the procedures become complicated.

The Bayesian randomization techniques can go one step further than just balancing the groups, the intervention and control. One can adjust the randomization to the outcome obtained. Of course, this requires the response to occur in a timely manner or a very delayed randomization process for study patient entry. These techniques are called “play the winner” or a “two-armed bandit”. In play the winner one randomizes to one intervention. If that is effective, keep randomizing to that intervention till it falls and then randomize to the other. This technique has created some strange outcome imbalances. The attribution of the success of one allocation arm may result from differences due to unforeseen factors that result in a distorted outcome. The first patient may be more severely ill, the intervention fails, and the next few patients may have milder illness and the intervention succeeds. The randomization occurs in one group direction due to less sick patients. This distorts the results. In the “two arm bandit” technique the probability of successful outcome is calculated after each randomization and one then adjusts the selection process to maintain a 50/50 randomization. Clearly the outcome must be known before the next patient is randomized which is not often possible in most studies.

Some Additional Thoughts

Randomization on a random basis is a very useful technique, especially when the intervention is blinded. It is important to state the techniques employed for randomization and how one maintains blindness in the methods section of the study publication. Years ago, if one was taking part in a multi-center study, one may have had randomization sequences in a sealed envelope assigning each patient’s allocation. This approach is mostly gone, first replaced by a telephone randomization system and now a computer-based system. The computer system can aid in determining patient eligibility, then using block randomization allocate the patient and inform the study management in which group to initiate the patient and replenish study supplies, usually form pre-positioned stocks. The central computerized randomization system facilitates quick accession of patients. A study site usually does not have a guaranteed allotment of patients and can be “shut out” of participation if it is not actively recruiting patients. However, the system can prevent a site imbalance with one site randomizing an excessive number of patients. Having one site dominate a study can significantly affect results. Finally, it is important to consider the timing of randomization. If a patient is randomized early in a study but the intervention starts days or weeks later, then the time period of randomization to intervention can provide an opportunity for multiple occurrences including death that can confound the study. How do you deal with a patient who dies after randomization, but before they receive treatment? Many advocate counting the patient as a failure (intention to treat) though clearly the outcome occurred without any relationship to treatment. We will discuss this problem in a later chapter. Suffice it is to say that randomization and treatment initiation should be tightly coupled in time to avoid this type of problem.

Chapter 9.
Participant Recruitment and Adherence

Recruiting study participants can be a difficult task. If the study involves patients that one sees often, and the patients are amiable to recruitment, accession of patients into the study will be successful. However, the inclusion and exclusion criteria can be so restrictive making recruitment impossible. One can be involved in studies where patients with the appropriate characteristics as outlined in the inclusion and exclusion are infrequently seen in one's medical practice. One can also work in an environment that is not conducive to research. Patients may be distrustful of research, or the institution may not support research endeavors. Obtaining sufficient study participants in these situations can be most difficult or impossible.

One consideration in recruitment is the optimal window for the science. A concept may be so new as to be unacceptable to colleague's or patients. As an example, that seems incredible now, hand washing in maternity wards was opposed by obstetricians in Vienna in the mid-19th century. Changing practice patterns may make referrals difficult and keep patients away from a study. A study evaluating patients with a patent foramen oracle (PFO), randomizing them to closure or not was a study that was very difficult to recruit patients because many cardiologists had made up their minds to close the foramen ovale, precluding referrals for the study. One can be faced with a situation with competing advances, where patients may be attracted to an alternative therapy. Physicians can also favor one approach over another diminishing referrals. Another problem affecting recruitment is an evolving medical practice and what is considered standard therapies. Because of changes in treatment, the disease state may change with outcomes significantly modified over the course of a 2-, 3- or 5-year study, making recruitment of the target population more difficult.

There are a number of reasons for a poor recruitment. One is the failure to start recruiting early. Waiting till all the study start up preliminaries are completed before identifying possible patients can be a costly mistake. This is especially true when one is involved in a multi-center study where the allocation of patients is on a "first come first serve basis". Organized centers on the day the study opens may have a large number of patients identified who can be consented and rapidly entered into the study. If one just expects patients to show up and colleagues to refer, one will probably fail due to inadequate recruitment. Being overly optimistic with insufficient recruitment planning will place a good study in jeopardy of failing.

Recruitment needs to be a constant effort throughout a study. Occasional surges in patients followed by pauses can adversely affect study efficiency, placing burdens on the study staff that could be avoided. Pressures build that can lead to inappropriate lowering of entrance criteria by the investigator or sponsor. While relaxing minor inclusion and exclusion criteria can be acceptable and helpful in recruitment, constantly trying to enter inappropriate patients may distort the study population and change the study outcome. In a heart failure study concerning arrhythmias, class IV heart failure was an exclusion. However, some sites persisted in trying to enter class IV patients by stabilizing them and then down classifying the patient's disease stage, leading to a distortion of the study since most of these patients with class IV failure initially, deteriorated early on so the arrhythmia endpoint could not be evaluated.

There are other factors that can make the study results less generalizable when changing entrance criteria. Failure to enter women or minority groups can make a study less generalizable. Do the results in white Caucasian males generalize to female, Hispanic or African American patients? Sometimes the lack of inclusion is due to the disease or the study location. VA centers tend to have mostly men. A heart failure study with ACE inhibitors carried out in Scandinavia will not likely have Hispanic or black patients. Thought needs to be given in the planning stage for site selection to avoid such situations of imbalance.

Recruitment Planning

One can plan to assess patients as they present to one's practice, clinic or when one is on service. Referrals can also be a means of obtaining patients. However, neither approach ensures a substantial availability of patients for a study. One should anticipate this and undertake backup planning. A record review can be useful identifying patients eligible for the study. Reviewing one's own files or obtaining permission to review clinic or hospital center files can be a useful resource in identifying patients who may be approached to enter the study. Needless to say, one needs IRB permission, appropriate HIPA consents in charts and agreement with colleagues who are the primary physicians for that patient.

Another approach is advertising for patients, especially advertisements in local papers, local radio and social media. All advertising must be reviewed by the IRB. One can give talks to physician groups, or hospital grand rounds to encourage referrals even more effective is to give talks to local groups of potential patients – YMCA's, senior centers, Shriner's groups, or rotary clubs, just to list a few groups that may have individuals or family members that could be interested in the study. Involving patient advocacy groups that are focused on the disease you are studying can be a great aid in patient recruitment.

Still recruitment may be difficult. The use of referral incentives can be helpful. In one study referral of 2 patients by a colleague earned the colleague a textbook of cardiology. If this does not work, involving colleagues at other sites or distant geographic areas may be advisable. Investigators involved in a number of studies can budget for a full time recruiter. This can greatly improve recruitment. One should not depend on any one of these strategies but utilize multiple strategies to insure adequate patient recruitment.

If one is uncertain as to the feasibility of recruiting patients into a study, one can consider a pilot study. The pilot study can be identical to the larger planned study. If the pilot shows that recruitment is feasible then the larger intended study can be undertaken. The pilot study can be a standalone, distinct from the larger, planned study (external pilot). An internal pilot study is one that when completed the results are to be combined with the planned larger trial. The internal pilot must utilize the same inclusion and exclusion criteria and have identical procedures to the definitive trial.

Recruitment feasibility is just one potential reason for a pilot study, but a very reasonable one to justify undertaking a pilot.

Recruitment Log

It is a good study practice to keep a recruitment log. A recruitment log may consist of:

Patient identifier

Sex

Age

Date of screen

Inclusion criteria (met or failed)

Exclusion criteria (met or failed)

Decision:

Entered

Excluded

Refusal by patient

A recruitment log or screening log can be very helpful for a number of reasons. The log can inform as to the reason for recruitment difficulties, as for example a number of patients being excluded for having one of the exclusion criteria. The log is also very helpful when trying to make the case that the study results are generalizable to the population at large. A review of the patient demographics can reveal some information as to generalizability. However, a study log adds additional information as to generalizability. When one sees in a paper that 5,000 plus patients were needed to recruit a hundred entered patients, this suggests a selected population being studied that is not generalizable. Perhaps the study's criteria for entry is too rigorous. Perhaps the exclusions are too limiting, excluding too many patients from consideration. If a large number of patients are excluded because they were "too sick", perhaps the study population does not reflect the severity of the condition being studied and the investigators are too cautious in entering truly sick patients. A recruitment log can help in understanding the type of patients studied and the possibilities that the population differs from what one might expect from patients with the disease. It would be very useful for published studies to present a summary of the recruitment log in an appendix of the study that can be accessed on-line.

Study Patient Adherence

Once recruited it is essential to keep patients in the study and adhering to the study protocol. Patients who fail to adhere to the protocol, who fail to show up on time for appointments and laboratory tests and who drop out of the study, do great harm. Dropouts can easily undermine a study, putting its outcome in question. If a patient drops out and is lost to follow up, the situation is even worse leaving the investigator with an unknown. Did the patient take the treatment and have a serious adverse reaction or found the treatment intolerable and dropped out of the study? Did the patient die from the treatment, but the event is unknown to the study investigators? These are questions that can't be easily answered and thus a diligent follow up, and systematic ascertainment of what happened to each patient is essential.

A 20% reduction in patient adherence to a study may result in the need to increase sample sizes by 50% to maintain the initial power estimate that led to the initial sample size calculation. A poor patient adherence is especially problematic in non-inferiority trials. With poor adherence the bias is to show no difference between the groups. If there is better adherence we might have seen a difference between the groups. The effect of excessive numbers of "dropouts" may result in a false positive result of non-inferiority.

One can try to increase patient adherence by planning ahead, making the study easier to follow, provide clear explicit directions and increased staff guidance to patients. Study duration should always be a consideration. The longer the study the greater the chance for patient dropouts given weather conditions. Permitting a range of visit times to allow for snowstorms and other severe weather is advisable. It's better to plan a simpler, easier to participate in study than a perfectly designed comprehensive project that doesn't take into consideration the limits of patient cooperation. It is also important not to recruit patients with the potential for poor adherence. Patients who are chronically unemployed, have addiction problems (narcotics, alcohol) or are disruptive should be considered potential problems and if possible avoided.

To improve adherence having an enthusiastic study team that is available to discuss issues with patients can go a long way to increase adherence. A 24/7 call in system for patients to have a response from study staff improves adherence and enhances patient safety. Having patients repeating instructions before leaving a visit and providing patients with instruction cards can also help. Patient call reminders for upcoming visits and laboratory tests are very effective. Recently apps have been developed to help a patient navigate a study reminding them about their medications and when visits are scheduled. This can be quite effective but many patients, especially over 50 find computer apps difficult to use. If a patient misses a visit or lab test immediate follow up is essential to avoid upsetting the study flow. Electronic reminders and compliance monitors such as medication supply bottle that confirms opening the drug container can be useful. In some trials where the concern with patient medication compliance is high the medications may be measured in blood or urine samples to verify compliance. A recent report of study medications being labeled so a quick scan of the GI system can ascertain treatment is going a bit too far and would be impractical to implement in most studies.

Periodic meetings between staff and patients, with updates provided on study progress can aid in adherence. Tracking adherence in the study tends to increase adherence. Displaying a chart of patient adherence increases the patient proclivity to adhere to the protocol. A frequently updated chart displayed in the study waiting room and consultation rooms can track group compliance on a monthly basis increasing study interest and participation. Counseling of non-compliant patients is important, and the investigators or study coordinators should meet with a patient to improve their compliance. Patients leaving the study need to meet with staff to ascertain the reason why and if appropriate discuss reasons for remaining in the study.

Adherence monitoring is an ongoing undertaking in any study. Early indication of poor study adherence should initiate a patient interview to see if modifications in study procedures are needed to increase study adherence. Pill counts may be a good indication of patient compliance, discrete questioning of patents to ascertain medication compliance is helpful. Visit adherence should be tracked and patients with poor adherence need to be contacted early by staff. Failure to keep appointments may place the patient and the study in jeopardy. Thought needs to be given to transportation. Can the patients afford multiple trips? Do they have assistance by family members if they can't travel on their own? Arranging for patient transportation may improve a patient's adherence to the protocol. Studies at academic medical centers where patients often travel considerable distance to reach the center recruit patients who can't easily return multiple times. This consideration needs to be discussed with the patient in the recruitment process. One constructive approach is for study sites to budget adequately for patient travel allowances that enable improved study compliance.

It is not always possible to ensure the recruitment of compliant patients or to convince a patient to remain in the study. For the study's integrity it is important to have the initial consent include provisions that permit the investigator to follow up with patients who drop out from the study. Permission granted in the initial consent is needed to contact the family, physician of record, hospital records or social security death records if need be. Obtaining outcomes such as hospitalization and death are important for study integrity as well as for the safety of all the patients being studied. It is critical to know if a patient drops out because of a serious side effect. A missing patient could be due to non-compliance or a death due to the therapy. This needs to be ascertained for the evaluation of treatments, and thus the safety of other patients in the study.

Chapter 10

Observational Studies

While some trialists discount observational studies and don't place them under the rubric of clinical studies, in fact observational studies are a critical part of clinical investigation. The association of smoking with lung cancer and the identification of critical risk factors for the development of coronary artery disease and atherosclerotic cerebral vascular disease are just some of the important contributions of observational research. While observational studies do not have the ability to determine causality as well performed randomized, blinded clinical trials, observational studies enable the medical field to develop insights into the relationships between characteristics or actions and outcomes. We could not randomize patients to smoking or non-smoking groups, follow the subjects for 10-20 years and see if they develop lung cancer. Could we randomize patients to high lipid diets, treated and untreated hypertension, high or low salt diets and follow the patients for decades to determine outcome. That can't be done in randomized, blinded trials but that information can be obtained and was using the technique of observational studies in Framingham, Massachusetts over the past 70 years (1948 to the present) as an example. The Framingham study was instrumental in showing the relationship between progressively higher lipid levels and coronary heart diseases, myocardial infarction, and death. The study among many important findings found hypertension to facilitate coronary artery disease, myocardial infarction, stroke, and heart failure. These observations led to clinical randomized, blinded trials to reduce myocardial infarction, stroke and death by reducing lipid (cholesterol) levels and treating effectively hypertension. The use of observational studies to identify potential risk factors to target in controlled, randomized, blinded studies with therapies has permitted the development of therapies and procedures underlying evidence based clinical medicine. The insights often develop first with cross sectional studies, followed by case-controlled studies and then cohort studies to cost effectively tease out the relationships of potential risk factors, noxious agents and adverse outcomes. Of course, there are many uses for observational studies, but in medicine we often see the paradigm of observational studies progressing to randomized, blinded controlled trials utilizing outcome measures.

Cross-Sectional Studies

Cross-sectional studies, sometimes called prevalence studies, look at both exposure and disease outcome at the same point in time. The investigative team both determines the exposure and disease's outcome simultaneously for each study subject. This study observes a subset of the population all at the same time, essentially a "snapshot in time" of the individuals exposed to a factor who has or does not have the condition being investigated. Since it's done all at once, we do not know if the exposure came before or after the disease. We do not have the ability to establish causation. What we can deduce is an association that may warrant further study. Besides the problem of not being able to establish a cause-and-effect relationship, there is the problem of survival. Since the cross-sectional study identifies all living cases at a given time, it selects out survivors. Others may have died before the evaluation so the relationship is between survivors who have the exposure or condition and the outcomes observed.

Case-Controlled Studies

A case-controlled study compares people with a condition, exposure or disease (cases) to those without the condition, exposure or disease. One can compare newly diagnosed cases (incident cases) to a control group, or one can compare all existing cases to the selected control group. With incident cases one needs to wait till they occur, which can take time. Taking all existing cases can save time, increase the pool of cases, but one has the survival problem as discussed with cross sectional studies. It may turn out that by using all cases one is selecting out for a factor that is more related to survival rather than exposure.

In a case-controlled study we determine what population of the control were exposed with their outcome and compare that to the population of cases exposed and their outcome. There will be exposed individuals in both groups, but where the exposed population has a greater risk from a given factor, it suggests that the factor plays a part in the disease process. Say 10 patients out of 100 in the control group has a high cholesterol, but 66/88 patents with a myocardial infarction have a high cholesterol. The report suggests high cholesterol increases the risk for a myocardial infarction. This is based on the comparison of the prevalence of risk factors in a group of patients with the disease compared to a group without the disease (controls).

Case control studies seem simple. Just identify case and select a control group, look for a difference and presto you have identified a contributor to disease, i.e., risk factor. However, the process is fraught with biases that can lead to some very wrong conclusions.

The areas that can cause difficulties are the selectin of cases, selection of controls, the "matching of the two groups" and the information obtained for the subjects based on recall. Recall is very variable and subject to bias. A patient with a disease, a condition causing distress is much more likely to possess recall than a person chosen as a control without an event.

Control Selection

Should controls selected represent the general population, or should they be very similar to the cases except for the disease or exposure? It depends on the situation. However, one does not want the control to introduce a bias. If the cases have coronary artery disease and the controls were screened or relatives of patients in a lipid clinic the selectin introduces a potential bias because of the potential genetic contributors to lipid abnormalities in the relatives of patients attending a lipid clinic. How controls are recruited can be an important factor. If one is studying hospitalized patients should controls also be hospitalized or should they be from the general community of non-hospitalized individuals? There is no clear answer to this question. Analyze the situation and try to remove as many possible confounding factors that could tie the control to the same underlying etiology as may be seen with the cases. Perhaps the best approach is to increase the control size to increase power and to have more than one control group. One can have multiple controls representing different groups to tease out potential confounders. Increasing numbers up to 4 controls for each case increases a study's power. Controls with multiple characteristics can help us avoid a characteristic (factor) that biases the study. By increasing the exposure in the control group of a relative causative factor can dilute the difference between the exposed and control groups. If risk is increased in one control group as compared to the case group, but not in other controls, then one may see a difference between different control groups and thus one needs to carefully evaluate the control group showing high-risk to see if there is a factor contaminating the selection process of controls. An example is a well reported study by Peal (Am J Hyg 9:97-159,1929) where the hypothesis that tuberculosis infection diminished the incidence of cancer. The controls were patients not dying of cancer in the hospital. It turned out that the control group of patients that did not die of cancer had more cases of tuberculosis, a common cause of admission to a hospital at that time. The conclusion of the study was that TB was protective against cancer. However, TB was a major cause of hospitalization in hospitalized patients that did not have a diagnosis of cancer. The factor that biases the observation was the frequency of TB in the hospitalized control population. A better control group would have been patients from the community that each cancer patient came from. It is likely that the incidence of TB would then be the same for both groups since they came from the same community.

Selecting cases can also have the problem that the relevant risk factor for the disease may be unique to a given group, region, or demographic. Selecting controls from multiple hospitals, multiple communities may help avoid this problem. The issue of incident or prevalent cases and selecting a survival factor if present may be a confounder. With prevalent cases one is dealing with patients (cases) that survived and they may not represent all cases, but rather the disease survivors and the factors that contribute to survival.

Matching

Another important consideration is how the cases and controls correspond to each other. Cases can be matched to controls for a number of factors except the factor that one is evaluating, that one suspects separates the cases from the controls. In this way the probability that the differences between the cases and control is due to selection of controls that are contaminated with characteristics that are associated with the factor under investigation can be reduced. One can match for age, race, gender, job, finances, or any number of factors. However, one must exclude matching for the factor that one suspects is the exposure or cause of the cases condition. One can match individuals, or one can match groups. Individual matching can be done in real time, while group matching is based on presenting characteristics and thus the cases need to be identified before the group can be constituted. Two possibilities then arise. We can study the cases vs controls for the matched characteristic or exposure, or if we match for a number of characteristics, it becomes more difficult to obtain controls as we increase the required characteristics that need to be matched. It becomes increasingly more difficult to find case with multiple matching characteristics that are required.

Establishing Exposure

In case-controlled studies the goal can be to establish the incidence of exposure in the cases versus controls. If the exposure occurs in the past few weeks that can be easily established. But if the exposure happened years ago, establishing exposure can be difficult. Memories can be very faulty especially if the exposure was of no consequence. However, if one develops cancer, gives birth to a child with a birth defect or develops a devastating neurologic disease, the suggestion that something may have precipitated the adversity can cause an intense such for a cause that can illicit false memories. Patients don't need a suggestion to introduce a bias, they often have searched their past memories for causation. This recall bias can greatly contaminate a case control study making it essentially useless. One also has the issue of the cases and controls correctly knowing the factual answer regarding exposure. Workers most often don't know the details of the chemicals that they work with. Patients often don't recall the diseases they suffered years prior or even a mediation taken years ago. Much recall can be guesswork. An investigator must be very careful to avoid leading questions; questions that put the exposure into the mindset of cases and controls. The best evidence for exposure is other than a person's recall. This need for interdependent confirmation of exposure can add considerable investigative work to ascertaining exposure in a case control study.

The advantages of a case control study are that it is inexpensive to conduct, simple to undertake, gives results quickly and is very useful with rare diseases or conditions that occur infrequently. The study can be perspective or retrospective. There are indeed some disadvantages as well. One can have a significant recall bias. One can't estimate the true incidence of a disease and one can introduce a factor in the selection of controls that can bias the findings of the study. One can have an indication bias where the outcome of interest may influence the exposure. An information bias where the outcome may affect the recollection of the exposure or a measurement bias where the occurrence may affect the measurement of the exposure. Often a case control study is performed to give direction to and support for the undertaking of a cohort study, which is more time consuming, costly and difficult to organize.

Case-Crossover Design

Cases are identified with a condition and an exposure is determined just before the case or event and contrasted to an exposure in the past not associated with the event. Thus, in this design the case serves as its control. One can design a trial where the cases were patients who had a cardiac arrest. The exposure could be the stress level on the morning of the arrest and a comparable time two months earlier. The problem would be to obtain an accurate assessment of the stress level at the distinct point in time, the control situation. Perhaps a more reliable study of this type would be patients with respiratory failure, looking at reported ozone levels on the day of a respiratory decompensation as contrasted to the ozone reported level at a distinct point in time. Since ozone levels are recorded daily in many localities, a reliable source would be available for the information, reducing information or recall bias.

Cohort Study

A cohort study starts with a population and follows them over time for outcome. It can begin with a general population or a defined population. The population may have already had the exposure of interest or the population over time may have the exposure in question. The exposure or the disease is not randomly assigned, but occurs in nature due to chance, patient characteristics, locality or an interaction of factors. The population studied, the cohort can be selected by geography, exposure, disease or defined by a set of pre-determined characteristics.

A cohort study can be perspective in that the cohort is selected and then over time the cohort has exposure and the disease can develop. The cohort can be followed for years, or even decades prospectively. Another approach is to have the cohort identified historically and then determine disease or exposure either contemporaneously or historically and subsequently follow prospectively as to outcome. This latter design can make a cohort study easier to undertake, one can obtain outcomes in a few years to a decade as opposed to a purely prospective cohort that can take far longer (decades).

A cohort study can be subject to the introduction of biases. In historical cohort study the information obtained for the group with the disease may be more robust than that for the group not having the disease. This information bias is somewhat like the recall bias seen in case control studies. It is important in a cohort study to have the critical information of disease, exposure and other relevant characteristics of the same quality and accuracy for the exposed as well as the non-exposed group.

Once individuals are identified in the cohort, their follow up is essential. Lost to follow up can be devastating to a cohort study as it is to a randomized trial. Analysis of cohort studies can be problematic. The investigator can introduce bias in the assessment of outcome. It is best to blind a cohort study analysis to exclude investigator and statistician introduced biases.

Cohort studies are most useful when the investigator already has an indication that the exposure can cause the disease and/or the characteristics of the population associated with the condition under study. Once the investigator has this understanding, the selection of the cohort can be more efficiently undertaken. The closer the temporal relationship is between the exposure and the disease, the easier it is to carry out a cohort study. Using historical data can make a cohort study more efficient. Cohort studies are time consuming and expensive to undertake. It is not an investigative program initiated lightly. If the investigator has little knowledge of the disease process, or the suspected duration of exposure that is associated with an outcome, one may need an extended observation period, making a cohort study less feasible. When conducting a cohort study, we need to ask if the results obtained in 10 or 20 years will still be relevant and worth the investment of funds and the time and effort of the study investigators.

Combined Observational Study Design

One combination is the case-control study initiated within a cohort study. A population is identified with baseline data obtained (through contemporaneous sources or historical information). The cohort is then followed in time for a period assumed necessary to develop the condition of interest. At a pre-determined time, the cases are identified as well as controls within the cohort who did not develop the disease. In a nested case control study from the cohort a control is selected at the time each case is identified, drawn from thc cohort. This enables the investigator to match the control to the case for the duration of follow up and for the time from initiating the cohort to disease identification in each case. Alternatively, when a case is identified in the cohort, a control is chosen at random also from the cohort. The control is not matched. This type of study is sometimes referred to as a case-cohort design.

The advantages of a combined design are a decreased cost because only the cases and controls in the cohort have their laboratory tests analyzed instead of the entire cohort. The data is obtained before the disease occurs and thus dependable and unbiased baseline information can be obtained. In these combined designs, the cases and controls are drawn from the same population and are thus less likely to have confounding factors contributing to disease development. The exposure that is more frequent in cases than in the control group is more likely to be the cause or a contributing factor to the disease development.

Summary

Observational studies are very useful tools. They don't result in the same high level of evidence that properly conducted randomized, blinded studies produce, but the information yielded by observation studies may be most informative. Often observational studies yield information that could not be obtained in a randomized, blinded trial design. While there are different levels of evidence obtained from different types of observational study designs, observational studies can be most helpful in addressing many clinical questions. Observational studies also obtain information that is critical to the design of controlled, blinded, randomized trials. For these reasons observational studies are critical tools in clinical research.

Chapter 11

Randomized Studies

The "gold standard" of clinical research is the randomized, blinded controlled study. It is the most reliable study design to reach a valid assessment of an hypothesis. However, even the randomized clinical trial can mislead due to the introduction of bias or the lack of adherence to the design plan.

An initial assessment of a clinical issue can be through a case series. This is where a clinician can assess a series of observations from cases to evaluate an outcome. Case series may be very useful to help describe the disease, be able to describe outcomes or assess potential risk. However, a case series can't establish causation and may often mislead as to the effect of a therapy because of the biases in case selection and hidden factors that can influence outcome. Thus, clinical studies that are designed to reduce bias and ensure comparable comparator groups are useful and a next step in the research process.

The selection of subjects needs to be such that groups being compared are similar, excluding factors that can influence the outcome other than the intervention under study. The best way to accomplish this is through randomization having the selection of group constituents established by chance. When making a comparison among groups, comparison of the intervention group to a control group can be made contemporaneously or have the control based on prior experience. Historic controls are easier to assemble, but they may introduce problems for analysis. The background therapies may have changed over time, and this could influence outcome, The disease may have changed, or the historic controls may represent a population with important differences from the intervention group currently being studied and this can affect outcome. For these reasons, it is best to perform the comparison of study groups constituted contemporaneously. But this may still lead to problems among groups being compared. If the population being allocated to the intervention or the control groups are not comparable as to factors that can affect outcome, then the study results may not be valid. Randomization of very large groups of subjects often yields comparable groups. But smaller studies of tens, or even hundreds of patients may not achieve balance. One can stratify the groups to make them comparable for known factors that may influence outcome. However, there are situations where the factors influencing outcome are unknown, limiting the usefulness of stratification. Also, if one stratifies the study into too many subgroups, statistical comparison of these small groups may be invalid due to the small size of each group. While there is no foolproof approach, it is best to undertake a study by undertaking a randomized, blinded, controlled trial to reduce bias as much as possible. Thus, the preferred study design is to have a control group and an intervention group created by randomization in which the investigator and the patients do not know which group received the intervention and which the control. This approach reduces bias as much as possible, produces comparable groups (especially when stratified) and meets the assumptions underlying the statistical tests we employ to evaluate the study data and then form conclusions.

The Parallel Study Design

The most basic study design is to compare a control group with an intervention over time, comparing the outcome in the two populations. If the two groups are comparable, the disease process in both groups is comparable with the only difference being the intervention a parallel study is most effective. However, if there are inherent differences between patients and these differences increase variability, comparing two or more groups over time with a parallel study design requires a larger sample size than the other common study design, the crossover study. In a parallel study one can study death as an endpoint since patients do not need to be re-allocated to the other intervention (treatment or placebo). Most parallel studies are done on top of standard therapy, reducing ethical problems an investigator may encounter in withholding standard of care therapies. With the parallel study one does not have to be concerned with a "carry over" effect as is the case with crossover studies since the subjects in each group stays on the therapy for a prescribed period of time without being exposed to the alternative therapy. The comparability of the groups and ensuring patient safety is dependent on the appropriate selection of inclusion and exclusion criteria for study entry.

The Crossover Study Design

An alternative to the parallel study design is the crossover study design. Each subject received both the intervention and the alternative (placebo or active therapy). Thus, each subject serves as his own control and thus since the comparison can be between each subject, this approach reduces inherent variability between subjects and thus less subjects are required in a crossover design for a comparable power. Sounds ideal, but there are many inherent problems with a crossover study design. The study assumes that the disease process is stable from the first arm of the study to the second arm. If the disease worsens over time, the second response may be different than those who receive active therapy in the first arm. This problem can be mitigated to a degree by randomizing the exposure of intervention or control as to which intervention is the first or second exposure on a random basis. Still this randomization design may not reduce the bias of disease progression. The study design falls if the disease is fatal during the study. One can't crossover a deceased study subject to receive the alternative exposure. One also has the problem of a "carryover" effect of the therapy in the alternative arm. There is usually a "washout" period between the two study arms, but that may not be adequate with some drugs. Amiodarone, an anti-arrhythmic drug with a half-life on average of 55 days when the drug is at steady state would make the duration of a crossover study prohibitively long. If a crossover design is selected, one should analyze for a period treatment effect. A crossover design is potentially useful in drug development when studying pharmacokinetics of a drug (oral vs. IV for example) or comparing two formulations (generic vs. a proprietary preparation) in patients with a stable disease or in normal volunteers.

The crossover design if it shows signs of difficulties with a carryover effect – a treatment period intervention, lack of disease stability, or a number of study "dropouts" at the time of being crossed over, can be converted into a parallel study by comparing the initial arms of the two groups in the study, one receiving the intervention first compared to the other receiving the control treatment first. Patients are randomized to the initial arm; it is blinded and the comparison of treatment to control arms can be accomplished similar to that done if the participants were in a parallel study. The possibility of a conversion of a crossover to a parallel study design should be specified in the study protocol, as well as the reason(s) why this analysis may be considered.

One approach to compensate for some of the deficiencies of a crossover design is to introduce a third period or randomly alternate study group sequences to reduce the effects of carryover, initial group randomization effect or potentially a placebo effect.

Factorial Design Studies

The factorial design is a more complicated parallel study looking at a number of interventions in a defined population. The factorial design compares a number of factors, say treatment A & B. One group will receive therapy A and a second group B. A third group would receive therapies A & B combined and a further group neither therapy A or B. When one makes multiple comparisons of A to B, A&B to no therapy and A or B to the combination therapy there is a decreased number needed in each group or "cell" of the study for the same power. However, the cell size may be too small for individual cell comparisons or sub-group comparisons, so the decision to employ a factorial design must be balanced between saving cost by reducing sample size and reducing the ability to perform multiple group assessments. The factorial study design is most useful when a pharmaceutical company is considering developing a combination product, combining drug A (the new drug) with an existing drug B, showing that the combination beats placebo (no therapy group). The study design can also show synergy when A & B is combined resulting in an effect greater than the effects of A or B alone.

Enrichment Studies

One can increase the chances of showing a positive outcome in a study by enriching the study population. Enrichment of the study population can be accomplished by only entering responders into the study. This can be done by having a "run in" period in the study where one needs to see a response to therapy before a patient is randomized. The run in is unblinded and then those who show a positive response are entered into the pool of patients who are then randomized to intervention or control. The problem is that the study results can only be generalized to patients who have been shown to respond to the intervention. A new blood pressure drug can be given to a patient, with an initial reduction in BP, the patient can be defined as a "responder" and then the results of the enrichment study can be generalized to other patient who initially responds to the therapy. Another approach to an enrichment study is to increase certain characteristics of the study patients as to increase the number of events in a study. In a COVID study I designed, only Hispanic and African American self-identified patients were entered, since both groups were reported by the CDC to have a higher morbidity and mortality to COVID-19 than the general population (twice the severity). The study was enriched with a higher at-risk population thus offering the possibility of a greater benefit in the treatment group. The study sample (number of patients) could be reduced while maintaining the desired 80% power.

Dose Titration Studies

Dose Titration Studies are often performed in a pharmaceutical development program early on to determine an optimum dose; optimum for efficacy or for safety or both. A group would receive one dose of a drug and then after a specified period of time a higher dose. The dosage amount can be in several increments with each dosing period being assessed with an efficacy metric and/or a safety outcome. A corollary of a dose titration study is a forced dose escalation study when the dose is increased at specified intervals for all patients till toxicity intervenes. Having all volunteers or patients receive increasing doses can increase risk for toxicity. The aim of the study is to find the highest effective dose that is tolerated by volunteers or patients. The dosing intervals are usually for weeks and the efficacy endpoints are ones that can be quickly determined, usually biomarkers are employed to determine effectiveness.

The initial dose in man is often based on pre-clinical animal studies. While in animals a full dose response curve is often explored, log range, in man the dose range explored is usually far less, ranging from dose x, 1.5x to 2x.

Withdrawal Studies

This study design aims at evaluation of duration of benefit of an intervention. Patients receiving a treatment can be randomly assigned to continue the treatment or stop the intervention. It is important to randomize the withdrawal of therapy to exclude a selection bias for selecting a group for cessation of therapy. The outcome may be that the treatment group maintains the observed effect and the withdrawal group shows a decline. This would support continued benefit of the intervention. This type of study is employed in pharmaceutical trials where after a pre-specified period of time patients are continued on the therapy under evaluation, unblinded or "open label". To determine if the therapy still shows activity over time a randomized blinded withdrawal of a fraction of the treated group can be conducted. This study design can give important information on the duration of therapeutic benefit after an initial response to therapy. The withdrawal study design can also evaluate a therapy that is often used but not established as effective. Often physicians are reluctant to enter patients into a randomized placebo-controlled trial to evaluate a therapy that may not be effective but one that is widely employed in the community. A randomized withdrawal is a viable alternative to evaluate if the therapy is effective. However, the withdrawal may not always show an immediate effect as in anti-hypertensive therapy. Stopping BP therapy does not always immediately lead to an early rebound in BP with a considerable percentage of patients maintaining BP control for months. Also, there may be a diminution of therapeutic benefit when the drug is re-introduced. It is believed by some experts that patients receiving L-dopa therapy who are abruptly stopped may not show as good a response on re-initiation of therapy. The patient should be informed of potential risks of a withdrawal study.

Unequal Allocation

For the parallel design study, the number of patients in each group may not be equal in numbers. More patients may be allocated to the intervention group to provide a greater number of exposures to therapy. Some investigators are concerned that this design compromises equipoise of the investigator. However, if the study is blinded, the intent of the study design to enhance exposure does not undermine the investigator equipoise. Rather it may offer a more rational allocation of resources.

Group Allocation

Instead of allocating by randomizing individuals into the arms of a study, one can allocate groups, communities, hospitals, or geographic regions. This can facilitate recruitment, especially in situations where individual allocation of an intervention is not possible. If one is evaluating the reduced infection rate with an air filtering system, individual patients could not be easily allocated. However, one could compare one hospital ICU with its air filtration system to another hospital without the newly introduced air filtration system. However, there could indeed be a problem of internal variability or with a factor associated with one group leading to competing outcome(s). What if the hospital with the new air filtration system has patients that are sicker with more varied or more severe pathology? The groups would not be comparable. One hospital could be a hybrid of a teaching hospital with referrals from community hospitals, as well as its own primary care patients. The other hospital could be a community hospital with a more homogenous population, perhaps less sick than the referral hospital. The outcomes could be very different between the two hospitals, regardless of the new air filtration system. One can also compare the hospital results with the new system to historic controls. However, there is a possibility that conditions have changed; the disease, the type of patients and the level of care between the older (historic) results and the results after the hospital has been re-fitted with the new filtration system. What if the re-fit coincided with a merger with a teaching medical center and the specialty care was augmented? Could this now affect outcome irrespective of the new filtration system?

Instead of randomizing a specific group with similar characteristics, all meeting study entry criteria one can randomize multiple groups with mixed characteristics forming a composite group all still meeting the study entry criteria. This is sometimes called cluster randomization trial; the cluster is more heterogeneous and thus more generalizable.

Equivalence Studies

The goal of this trial design is to show that two therapies are similar within a specified margin and thus by the parameters set in advance are equivalent. While most trials are intended to show superiority, an equivalence study aims to show similarity. Choosing the margin often is controversial. In the pharmaceutical industry a trial to establish a generic drug's equivalence to a brand drug (originator) is done using margins set by FDA between 80 – 125% of the drug's bioavailability. Thus, to be equivalent the generic drug must show levels in an in vivo bioavailability study no less than 20% of the mean drug level and no more than 25%. In other equivalency studies the selection of the equivalence margin is up to the investigator. A margin of 20% is generally considered reasonable. Some argue one should consider up to a 50% margin, but that would be considered excessively wide margin by many, since the margin of an effect size benefit is usually in the 20% range at most. Setting a margin that will be accepted by most people evaluating the study is difficult. Setting the margin too wide will make the study results unacceptable, while a very narrow margin may make the study less likely to show equivalence.

When considering an equivalency trial there are a number of important considerations. The study population should be similar to that in the trial that established the efficacy of the therapy. If the trial shows the agent to be effective in mild to moderate hypertension, then a trial undertaken to show similar efficacy of another agent in a hypertensive population should evaluate mild to moderate hypertension. Comparing the established therapy to the new therapy under investigation in a population with resistant hypertension would not be appropriate and would not necessarily lead to the conclusion that the therapy under study has effects that are equivalent. If the two therapies had the same effect, one could not conclude that the agents were effective, If they both failed to affect BP in the resistant population one could not conclude that they were ineffective. Perhaps any study in this population would show no affect, in other words the study would not have assay sensitivity. So, a similar population, a similar disease, and similar concentration achieved are needed. A consideration that can lead to study “manipulation” is choosing a less potent dose for the comparator than that studied in other trials showing efficacy and comparing it to a more potent dose of the intervention under study. This can manipulate (bias) the outcome of a study. Another problem is sample size estimation and event rate. The sample size is dependent on the event rate to show a significant difference or to establish equivalence or non-inferiority. If the estimated event rate turns out to be lower that predicted as is often the case, then the preset equivalency margin can be too wide, making the study claim of equivalence subject to dispute.

Non-Inferiority Studies

A non-inferiority trial is very frequently employed in clinical research. Given the number of therapeutic interventions that are considered effective, as well as physician reluctance to employ placebo therapy for serious disease states, more and more clinical research employs a non-inferiority design to compare a new therapy to an established one. This is especially the case when the new therapy can't be added to standard therapy. An example is the use of the combination drug of sacubitril – valsartan (Entresto®) that is a neprilysin inhibitor combined with an angiotensin II receptor inhibitor. One can't study this drug on top of an angiotensin receptor blocker, or an ace inhibitor because one may obtain excessive hypotension or exacerbate a toxicity, angioedema. Thus, because of safety concerns the efficacy of this agent was established by a study comparing an angiotensin receptive inhibitor to the combination drug (Entresto®). The study had a superiority margin set as well as a non-inferiority margin. Similarly, the comparison of a new anticoagulant to warfarin could be set up as a non-inferiority trial. The novel anti-coagulant (NOAC) and warfarin may be equally effective, but the novel agent may cause less bleeding and be more convenient to take without having to surveil bleeding times with multiple blood samples. One could not treat a group with placebo for comparison and one could not combine a NOAC with warfarin.

In a non-inferiority trial, the confidence margins are critical in establishing significance for non-inferiority. So, if the trial is messy, has a lot of noise, a lot of variability, or a significant number of non-compliant patients, these factors would increase variability and thus there is an overlap in the confidence intervals of the agents being compared and non-inferiority may be claimed. However the similarity in outcome of the two groups would be factitious , a study with wide confidence intervals, or with the mean differences in outcomes decreased more than was expected (with the non-inferiority margin unchanged) would yield findings that are rejected by most researchers as having failed to establish non-inferiority.

The approach for analysis of a non-inferiority study starts with a point estimate and a confidence interval. We can obtain an estimate of the relative risk of the intervention compared to the control. We can estimate a point where the relative risk of the two interventions is equal to one (the identity point). From then we can establish the non-inferiority margin (delta). If the point estimate of efficacy of the drug in question, as well as the upper 95% confidence interval margin of the relative risk is less then one, the intervention is superior (A). If the confidence interval around the point estimate crosses one, the point of identity, but the upper margin of the confidence interval is less than delta, the result is non-inferior (B). If the confidence interval crosses one, but the upper margin of the confidence interval is greater than delta, the finding is non-inferior (C). If the lower margin of the confidence interval is greater than one and the upper margin of the confidence interval is greater than delta, than the intervention or drug under study is inconclusive (D). If the point estimate is less than 1 and the upper margin of the confidence interval is greater than delta then the drug under study is inferior (E). This can be seen in figure I adapted form Pocock and Ware (Translating study findings into plain English, Lancet 200,373:1926-1928).

Figure I. Non-Inferiority Study Results

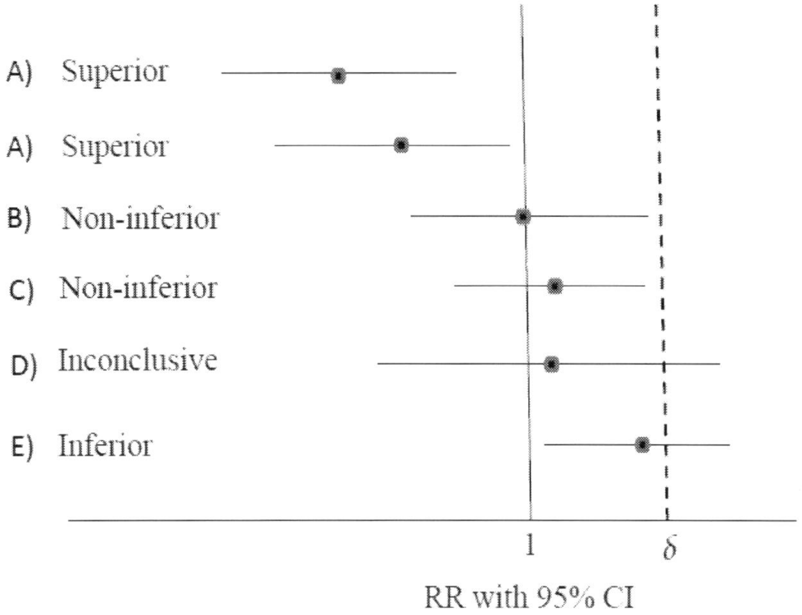

How one analyzes the trial can be critical. If one uses the intention to treat analysis paradigm, then patients not on therapy or receiving the alternative therapy are counted and the results favor a non-inferiority outcome. Increased variability (noise) will also favor a non-inferiority outcome. For a non-inferiority study, one should use an “on treatment analysis”. To do otherwise increases the chance of a false positive non-inferiority outcome. Another issue is the sample size, one that is too small would favor a negative outcome in a superiority trial, not enough power. However, in a non-inferiority trial an inadequate sample size would lead to not showing a difference and thus establishing non-inferiority. This again would yield a false positive outcome.

Non-inferiority studies appear simple but can be "tricky" and can mistakenly yield a non-inferiority claim when in fact the outcome is due to methodologic mistakes, not non-inferiority.

Behavioral Trials

A behavioral trial aims to modify a behavior that might be a risk factor contributing to an unwanted outcome. The investigators target a behavior that may be modified and by so doing affect outcome. The intervention can modify behavior of an individual compared to individuals without the intervention, or it can modify group behavior and compare outcome to a group who did not receive the behavioral intervention. This approach is different than what usually occurs since by taking part in the study a subject's behavior is modified and the modification is evaluated as to its change in the clinical outcome. The behavioral intervention can and should be blinded just as a drug or surgical procedure can be blinded.

Large Simple Clinical Trials

Clinical trials have become very complex, evaluating many endpoints with large numbers of patients studied. The process is very time consuming and costly. An approach to reduce cost is to simplify the study, reduce time and effort of study personnel, but still affording critical insights is the large simple trial. The trial tries to evaluate outcomes that can be documented easily in a large population. The large population helps distribute confounders equally amongst the study groups. The trial omits detailed characterization of the population being studied. Given the size of the trial it can easily be generalized to the therapeutic target population. Studying less complex response variable works best in the “simple trial” with mortality or hospitalization as favored endpoints. Laboratory tests are kept to a minimum or omitted from the trial completely. While the trial may be blinded at times it may be an open label with the expectation that the large number studied makes up for the lack of blinding. With its vast number of patients, the impact of bias with an unblinded trial is reduced. Follow up is critical since the success of the trial is determined by the endpoints being obtained. Sometimes the number of potential interactive patient characteristics that can confound outcome are daunting and even a large simple trial may potentially fail. In these situations, the “mega trial” involving tens of thousands even hundreds of thousands of participants becomes an alternative. Such large trials are so large as to have the population approach the population that one intends to generalize to. However, the mega trial can have its flaws when a large but still homogenous population is to be recruited. Including all those in a population of Norway, Denmark and Sweden still would not result in a patient population with characteristics that are generalizable to a diverse population as we see in the United States. An example of the simple trial was the evaluation of beta blockers post MI. Patients were randomized to receive the drug (beta blocker) or placebo and followed for a year to determine the effect of drug therapy on survival. Physicians in the community were given postcards to report entry of a patient into the study and then follow up was obtained to determine outcome in a year’s time. It helps to have a national database recording all deaths to verify outcome. If the follow up post card in the mail arrives (which in the U.S. these drugs may not be the case) one can fall back on a death registry. Still this simple design provided important therapeutic information. Beta blocker therapy post myocardial infarction these past forty years has saved the lives of millions of patients worldwide. However, the drawback of these studies is the minimal information provided often precluding subgroup analysis or the development of new therapeutic hypothesis for further analysis of the study database.

Run-in Studies or Pilot Studies

A run-in study can be used to assess the potential for compliance of patients in a planned study. It can also be useful to identify respondents to a therapy and thus can be employed in the selection of patients for entry in an enrichment trial. A pilot can be used to train staff and determine the feasibility of a study, determine if recruitment is feasible or, testing procedures are effective in the assessment of study endpoints. A pilot can be an external pilot where the pilot study is separate from the main study. Alternatively, a pilot can be an internal pilot where the study results are incorporated into the larger study with the definitive study as an expansion of the pilot. An internal pilot is most advisable since the time, effort, and costs to obtain the pilot data can be incorporated into the main study. Nothing is wasted and the risk patients accept to be in the pilot is balanced by the benefits of the outcomes obtained that are incorporated into the larger study that has the power to reach a definitive conclusion. Incorporating the results of the internal pilot with the definitive study must be pre-specified for the process to be statistically valid.

Delayed Start Design

An intervention may modify the population, changing outcome even if the intervention is transitory. One approach of evaluating this is the delayed-start design. One can first evaluate the intervention as compared to the control group as to an outcome measure. Then all the patients are placed on the intervention and evaluated as to the diseases modifying effects. One can contrast the outcome of those who received active treatment first vs those who received the control therapy and then active treatment. Did first receiving active therapy change outcome observed in such a study? There are questions that the delayed study start design can address.

Platform Studies

This is a logistical design facilitating multiple studies on a similar topic. A group of centers have staff that can undertake certain disease focused studies and the research group has a ready supply of patients. Many of the evaluation, recruitment and follow up procedures are similar among planned studies and can be facilitated by establishing a platform to undertake future studies. The research coordination creates a platform to study a particular condition, facilitating a clinal trial start. As new treatments, procedures, therapies come along the organization or consortium has a “platform” to rapidly initiate clinical trials in the areas to be studied with proficiency. This can be a very useful and important methodology. COVID-19 identified a great deficiency in the world research establishment. There was no ready mechanism to undertake controlled, randomized, blinded trials on existing drugs to see if those agents offered possible benefits. Instead of arguing in the press the potential efficacy of hydroxychloroquine, early steroid therapy, anti-platelet drugs or other possible interventions there should have been a "platform" available to initiate trials to rapidly obtain results based on randomized clinical trials.

The N of 1 Study Design

Given a therapy to a patient and reporting the outcome would be a case study. However, one can expand the utility of this approach by administering a therapy or control treatment in a random way, repeatedly to a patient. Clearly the outcome must be easily assessed in a short period of time and the outcome can't be a severe morbid or mortal event, prohibiting repeating the intervention or the control intervention. By varying the intervention (therapy or control) allowing time for washout of drug effect and allowing for the patient to return to a baseline state, one can assess the difference between control and intervention effect. One can assess the patient - treatment interaction in an N of 1 study. This type of study diminishes the variance in response to repeated therapeutic interventions. The same person is being treated thus reducing the inter – individual variability. One then can expand the study to combine multiple "N of 1" studies, each in an individual patient. In combining multiple exposures, one can assess the variation between patients and the variation within a patient. The effect can be measured excluding a good deal of variability with a small number of patients. The generalizability of such a study is limited due to the small number of patients exposed.

Multi-Center Trials

The multi-center trial has been developed to enable the recruitment of adequate numbers of patients. The multi-center trial has become ever more important as investigators have employed power calculations that show that a large number of patients are needed to have an adequate power to statistically determine a true positive outcome and reject the null hypothesis. Multi-center trials also reduce imbalances between the intervention and control groups by having patients recruited from multiple centers making for a heterogenous population and thus insure a better representation of the general population. By having multiple investigators, the possibility that investigators interject bias into the study or tamper with the outcome becomes less impactful on the study outcome. Multi-center studies may help adjust for variations in regional practice patterns that could influence study outcome. However, with international multi-center study medical practice could be so varied as to confound outcome and thus adversely affect the studies interpretation. Similar baseline therapy and patients with a consistent disease state need to be studied at all centers in a study. While the basic design of a multi-center study is the same as a single center; parallel or crossover, the organization needed to manage a multi-centered study is far more complicated.

There is usually an organizing committee that initially plans the study, recruits, participant investigators, provides study management, assists in the study close out, supervises data analysis, study result publication and the reporting of results to relevant parties – investigators, participants, and sponsor(s). Some studies besides a planning committee have a coordinating center to manage the trial, establish central core laboratories, replace and recruit new investigative sites, operate the randomization system, collect the study data and coordinate the statistical analysis. Most multi-center studies have a data safety monitoring board (DSMB) to follow study outcome contemporaneously to ensure patient safety. The organizing or planning committee will arrange for IRB initial and continuing approval. The IRB also approves study recruitment advertising and the proper monetary amount of a patient honorarium. Very large studies may also have a body representing investigators, an "Assembly of Investigators". Many of these large multi-center trials are financed by the NIH, NCI, or the pharmaceutical industry and can cost in the hundreds of millions of dollars. Clearly these types of studies are not initiated on a whim but are the culmination of many supporting studies looking for a definitive, often natural history outcome.

Still some multi-center trials are failures. Magnesium was believed to possess anti-arrhythmic properties, reducing sudden death. In vitro studies supported magnesium's anti-arrhythmic action. A large observational study and a meta-analysis of smaller randomized trials showed clinical benefit for magnesium therapy. However, a very large multi-center study found no benefit for magnesium. A drug in development by Pfizer Pharmaceuticals that raised high density lipoprotein (HDL) had early promising results with surrogate markers for coronary disease risk, but a large Phase III study showed no benefit in survival and in fact an adverse outcome. Large multi-center trials have become the "gold standard" for evidence based medical practice and at times required for regulatory approval of pharmaceutical therapy. However, just being large does not ensure success or reliability of finding a definitive outcome.

Mega Trials

One type of large multi-center study is the mega-trial involving 10,000 or more patients. The mega trial is not a large simple study, but a carefully designed intensive trial, almost invariably a parallel study design, with large numbers of patients to test a therapeutic hypothesis, or to reveal a low frequency adverse event. The trials may be sponsored by the pharmaceutical industry to develop "blockbuster" drugs that are intended to treat millions of patients with chronic diseases with the treatment intended to last decades. These trials are very costly, but given the revenue obtained by blockbuster drugs, "billion dollars" a year or more annual revenue for these treatments the trials are easily justified on a future earnings.

The Clinical Registry

A clinical registry can be analogous to a single intervention arm of a study. A registry usually does not have a control group, it lacks a comparator. However, the registry has a defined population with inclusion and exclusion criteria with consent obtained and with prescribed patient follow up. Often and especially in the medical device field, a margin is established by consensus as to what the benefit margin might be, to be able to state that the intervention was non-inferior or superior to an established performance expectation. Clearly, the registry design is more than a case series, but is it a valid study? Some believe it is useful to follow exposure to an intervention to obtain safety information, while others believe it an effective design to establish efficacy. The difficulty is establishing the metrics for a performance standard and making the "leap of faith" to the use of a performance standard as contrasted to a comparator trial that has an alternative or no treatment group is a difficult one. The registry is indeed a very effective way to obtain follow up on an intervention in patients treated outside of the rigors of a clinical trial, who are treated in the community. It is effectively used by FDA for "real world" exposure experience, post approval. The trouble with a registry is that many device developers propose to use the registry as a means of determining efficacy and thus the basis of approval. This is highly speculative and lacks data supporting this approach, perhaps a "bridge" too far.

Comparative Effectiveness Studies

These studies compare a new therapy, often a drug to alternative therapies both in terms of efficacy, safety, as well as costs. For drug approval in Europe, comparative studies are usually required, but not in the U.S. Since it may not be in a pharmaceutical company's interest to sponsor studies of its therapy vs. a competitor, especially if there are both compared at optimum effective doses, the NIH at congressional direction has taken on the sponsorship of many important comparative effectiveness studies. While not glamorous, these studies can be the “backbone” supporting clinical practice and formulary decisions, and support the practice of evidence based medicine.

An Overview

Looking at clinical trials from the objective of a clinical trialist, studies can be exploratory or pragmatic. An exploratory trial would be one where one aims to elucidate a biologic process. A pragmatic trial may be one aimed to determine a better or safer treatment. In an exploratory trial the target is to answer a mechanistic question. Thus, one wants the population to be as homogenous as possible to avoid confounders. One is looking for a specific mechanism or biologic target to affect. One wants to maximize treatment effect by giving the highest tolerated dose of a therapy. The protocol would require rigorous subject supervision and monitoring. The control group usually receives placebo (to maximize the difference in effect size) and the analysis should be an “on treatment” analysis to reduce the noise contributed by study “dropouts”, or study “drop ins”. On treatment analysis reduces variability and results reflect the direct effects of the drug or therapeutic approach being evaluated.

Pragmatic studies are treatment directed. They should recruit a heterogenous population. The study is aimed at a pragmatic determination of what therapy is effective and what therapy is ineffective, not to determine a mechanistic understanding. The study aims at finding a therapeutic intervention effective in in a very broad segment of the population. The dose one chooses aims to be effective but avoids serious or bothersome side effects. The determination of efficacy is assessed with less intrusive measurements, that make the study easier to carry out. Instead of a placebo the study usually compares the intervention to standard of care therapy and the observation period is often longer than in a mechanistic study. In pragmatic studies the preferred analysis is "intention to treat", but for drugs that cause side effects causing large numbers to drop out "on treatment analysis" may be informative as to efficacy and the AE rate and "drop out" number inform as to tolerability and therapeutic adherence. Thus, both an intention to treat and an on-treatment analysis should be performed.

Regardless of the intent of the study it is important to select effective metrics to evaluate outcome using the best available technologies. The use of biomarkers may be helpful though they may not always relate to morbid/mortal outcomes. To reduce sample size which translates to a reduction in cost and reduced difficulty in completing the study, one wants to maximize the treatment effect and minimize variance. Comparing a drug to placebo requires a smaller sample size than a comparative study that may require an increase of 4 to 8 times in sample size. One should strive to decrease variance in a study. Controlling for and reducing the influences of covariates reduces variance and biases. Using patients as their own control as is the case in a crossover study can help reduce confounders and variance, reducing sample size as long as the treatment effect can be “washed out” in a reasonable time and that the disease is stable for the duration of the study. By introducing outcome measure with greater precision one can also reduce variability. When outcomes are assessed by questionnaires, making the measurements more frequently and/or using multiple scales, can increase precision and thus diminish variability.

Many times, subjects who enter a study are at the peak of their illness or in a period of escalation of disease severity. That is when patients present for medical care and are then entered into a study. As time passes the patients continue in the study symptoms may tend to subside for both the treated and the non-treated groups. This phenomenon is often called “regression to the mean”. One can often avoid this issue and identify the problem by including a no treatment group. Alternatively, a “cooling off period” if the disease state being studied permits, may be helpful in not recruiting patients at (or near) the height of the disease process avoiding the regression of symptoms severity as time passes.

In placebo controlled studies there are cautions needed. A placebo is not always the “magic bullet” for a study. Patients tend to shy away from placebo-controlled studies and placebo can be identified by subtle cues that the patient perceives that may identify active therapy. One can subtract the placebo effect from the intervention effect to determine the true effect and thus quantify the placebo effect. One can be misled in that the placebo effect can be mistaken for patients who symptoms are subsiding (regression to mean), which can enhance the effect size of the intervention. Having a "cooling off" period for disease stabilization and then a placebo "run-in" may optimize, allowing for "regression to mean" and the placebo effect. Placebos can be identified from active therapy in some studies. A study evaluating Vitamin C vs. placebo, the placebo did not have an acidic taste thus differentiating the placebo from the treatment. Studies with IV infusion with the active treatment causing irritation at the infusion site or a feeling of warmth can reveal the active treatment. One can attempt to avoid this unmasking by employing an "active placebo", a placebo that has some of the identifying characteristics of the active treatment, essentially misleading the patients and maintaining study blind. At times the treatment method of administration may be so different from the comparator making blinding difficult. Comparing an IV drug to a pill is an example. One can still blind by using the "double-dummy" technique. One can administer the active IV treatment and an inactive pill (placebo) compared with the active pill and an IV placebo. In this way the blind can be maintained.

Careful thought and planning is requisite in the study design choice and its execution to maintain study integrity. In designing a clinical trial one needs to focus on the study question, optimizing all aspects of the study to answer the primary study question in a fair, unbiased way.

Chapter 12.
Quality of Life Measurements and Economic Impact Studies

When one is designing a trial for a new drug, a new treatment, a new procedure, or new diagnostic, it is useful to evaluate the cffcct of thc intcrvention or quality of life and its economic impact as well as its safety and effectiveness. Some trials are designed as quality-of-life assessments or economic impact evaluations as standalone trials. However, if the primary endpoint is an effectiveness measurement, quality of life or economic input can be a included as a secondary endpoint. This is rather straight forward and can be exceedingly useful.

Quality of Life Measurements

A study evaluating participant quality of life can be greatly affected by the underlying disease state. Measurements of quality of life needs to take into account the condition and the specific effects of the disease. Quality of life measurements need to be multi-dimensional, evaluating differing aspects that affect quality-of-life. Some dimensions to consider are physical functioning, psychological factors, social functioning, personal satisfaction, and the individual's perception of health status. Some additional dimensions such as cognitive ability, physiological function, personal productivity, intimacy, sexual fulfillment, and quality of sleep can be considered. An evaluation may not cover all these dimensions, depending on the disease state, the areas that the treatment may affect (both positively and negatively), as well as the goal of undertaking the evaluation. A treatment targeted to improve mobility in a condition due to a muscular skeletal physical injury would probably not include an evaluation of cognitive ability.

Physical function may evaluate activities of daily living or the ability to initiate a physical exercise program. Social function may involve the subject's ability to interact with family, friends, community and if the patient can fulfill his social obligations. Psychological functioning can entail the subject's emotional well-being, the extent of anxiety, despair, guilt or worry. The patient's emotional state should be evaluated whether it is a positive or negative. One can also ascertain the subject's degree of satisfaction, the extent of the perception of overall well-being.

It is important to determine the perception of health status. This may differ considerably from the subject's true health status. Often the subject's perception correlates best with the subject's eventual outcome. In a quality-of-life assessment one can evaluate the change in the subject's disease and how it effects the patient's perception of quality of life, change in a patient's functional status and the degree to which the subject's life has been influenced by the disease and its progression.

When measuring the quality of life in a clinical study, there are a number of considerations to take into account. The instrument measuring the quality of life should not be an undue distraction from the study procedures and compliance with treatment. Personnel evaluating the quality-of-life question must be trained and the procedure standardized. The extent of the questioning is a consideration. How it is presented and what cognitive level is required to respond needs to taken into consideration. Additional considerations are the study population's age, sex, language skills, culture, as well as cognitive abilities.

Timing of when the questions are to be administered is important and can greatly affect results. A baseline is essential. Enough time is required for the intervention to take effect, but too long an interval may permit the progression of the disease to dominate the reported effects. In a heart failure evaluation with an ace inhibitor therapy questioning the patient as to quality of life in the first few weeks may not reveal any effect of treatment in subjects with severe heart failure. It may take a month for the treatment to show an effect. The time course of treatment effect may be an important finding.

The approach to obtaining information from patients can affect the results obtained. One can use a telephone-based questionnaire. This can be anonymous and elicit answers that would not be readily volunteered in person. "On-line" is the modern alternative but requires patient access to a computer and the ability to participate in the study online. The responses of patients may be less reliable, and participation may be erratic. Face-to-face interviews are more reliable but are time consuming and costly. Patients may not reveal intimate details in a face-to-face interview. However, when combined with a patient's scheduled visit, face to face interviews are more likely to be completed. Self-administered questionnaires have more missing data but may contain more intimate responses. Self-administered questionnaires may also have the drawback of obtaining a group response or that of a caretaker and not reveal the patient's true feelings.

The frequency of assessment needs to be considered. Does one aim to evaluate an acute or a chronic effect or both? Should one evaluate at each point in a study when there is an adjustment or change in the therapy or a change in dose of the treatment. If a patient shows signs of disease progression or a "relapse" is there a process to re-evaluate the quality-of-life measure?

Instrument Selection

There are a large number of instruments to choose from. There are generic instruments, or condition specific instruments. There are population specific instruments. Some instruments measure a condition for a specific disease while others can be utilized in a multi-disease state. Some focus on a specific health profile while others evaluate general health or an improvement in health status. One can administer a single questionnaire, or a battery of instruments covering a single or multiple dimensions. Administering a battery of tests or one test multiple times measuring a specific aspect of health may increase the precision of the measurement, decrease variance and thus reduce the number needed to study for a given effect size and a specified alpha (prespecified margin of success).

Some of the generic instruments to consider are the SF-36, EQ-5D, Rotterdam Symptom Check List, Mental System Assessment Scale or the NIH PROMIS System. In the pediatric area there are age specific general scales such as PedsQL, Kids SCREEN and PROMIS instruments. Then there are specific instruments depending upon the area of study. For psychology there is the CDRS-R for depression, the Patient Health Questionnaire (PHQ), the Profile of Mental State (POMS) and the Centers for Epidemiological Studies Depression (CES-D) instruments.

For cancer studies there is the Assessment of Cancer Therapy (FACT), European Organization for Research and Treatment of Cancer Quality of Life (EORTC QLQ). The Barthel Index, a measurement of physical function and independence can be employed in physical training studies. For heart failure studies the Minnesota Living with Heart Failure Scale is often employed, or the Kansas City Cardiomyopathy Questionnaire, or Heart QoL – European Society of Cardiology questionnaire.

Utility Measurements

Utility measurement assess preferences and can also be called preference scoring. These measurements evaluate a patient's preferences for outcomes related to morbidity and mortality. The outcomes can be quantified with a unified score, a single weighted measure with the quality of adjusted life (in years) called the QALY. This can yield the sum of the benefits less the negatives of adverse effects with an increasing disease burden.

This measure can be employed in a semi-quantitative assessment as the basis of a cost utility analysis. This type of analysis may be helpful in evaluating two or more competing interventions.

One can assign a numerical value to a series of outcomes. Often death is assigned 0 and normal complete health 1. Intermediate assessments can be compiled by a "trade off" method where a participant can choose an outcome that they would want and be willing to take the risk of death to obtain.

Pharmacoeconomics

One of the areas where utility analysis is often used is in pharmacoeconomic assessment of pharmaceutical products that are being compared. A pharmacoeconomic study evaluates the cost expressed in monetary terms and the effect (efficacy or quality of life) of the treatment expressed in monetary terms. One can evaluate direct costs (price, staff expense, capital expended); indirect costs (loss of earnings, loss of productivity, cost of product development). One can evaluate benefits in terms of life years saved, utility units (quality and quantity of life) mobility and psychological as well as social outcomes can also be evaluated in this way.

Cost Minimization Analysis

This analysis compares the monetary cost of different therapeutics that have similar health outcomes. The comparison is based on cost.

Cost Effectiveness Analysis

This technique analyzes two or more therapies that have the same treatment objective but may have different degrees of effectiveness. The question becomes how much additional benefit is obtained by one therapy as compared to the incremental cost to obtain a "better" or a lesser but satisfactory outcome. This approach calculates the incremental cost of a therapy comparing therapy A to therapy B to obtain the incremental cost effectiveness ratio (ICER):

$$ICER = \frac{\text{Cost A} - \text{Cost B}}{\text{Effect A} - \text{Effect B}}$$

The selection of the effect measurement and its magnitude is based on the clinical assessment made by the investigator. The more quantitative the measurement can be the greater the reliability of the assessment.

Cost Effectiveness Diagram

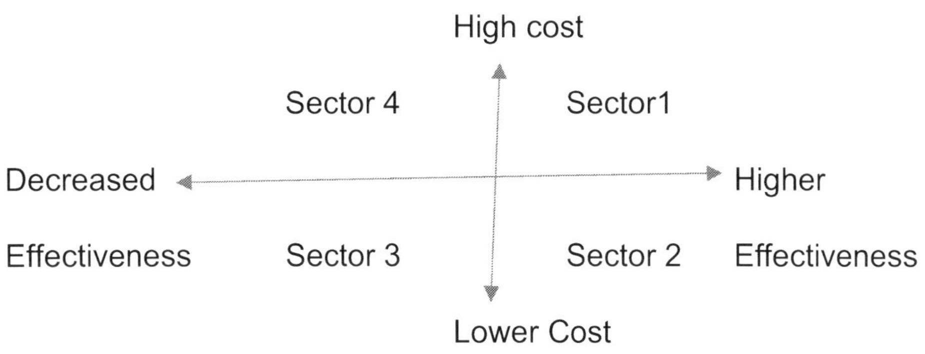

Sector 1 higher effectiveness with higher cost
(a health care decision)

Sector 2 higher effectiveness and lower cost
(ideal)

Sector 3 lower cost and lower effectiveness
(sub-optimal but may be a decision made of economic necessity)

Sector 4 lower effectiveness and higher cost
(Unacceptable but may still be pushed by a marketing group)

Cost Utility Analysis

Compare costs to quality and quantity of life. The measure most commonly used is a quality adjusted life year (QALY). This can offer a more complete picture of the cost benefit assessment since both the quality and quantity of life are considered. As an example, if one determines that a treatment results in a quality-of-life weight of 0.6 per years. Then if the patient lives 4 years the QALY improvement will be 0.6 x 4, or 2.8 QALYS. Thus, an instrument can compare the standard treatment to a newly introduced or alternative treatment a 2.8 vs. 1.0 quality would be a substantial improvement.

Besides QUALYS there are DALYS, or disability adjusted life years. This can be used to measure the overall burden of disease by combining death and disability into one measurement, years of life lost plus years lived with a disability.

Cost Benefit Analysis

Both cost and benefits are measured in monetarily terms (in dollars). The cost of a life is often set at 2 million dollars for insurance purposes. One then compares the cost of the treatment to the monetary amount estimated to be added to the life expectancy. One can estimate each additional year of life at $28,571 if life expectancy is set at 70 years and is equal to 2 million overall. If a treatment increases life by 2 years, or $57,143 and costs $70,000 one can consider the societal cost appropriate. What is the point at which a treatment is considered too expensive based on a cost benefit analysis is a most difficult question to address. However, cost benefit analysis is an effective technique in posing these difficult questions.

Chapter 13

Adverse Event Reporting

An adverse event is a clinical occurrence, physical sign or symptom that is unwarranted. An adverse event can be expected or unexpected. They are often unpredictable and may occur in the treated or untreated study group. Studying adverse events occurrences is usually not the intent of a study though some studies do set out to show fewer adverse events in one group than another. Unlike the primary outcome, a difference in adverse event frequency is usually not powered for in a study. Given the small size of most studies adverse events are not evaluated statistically with the frequency of adverse event occurrence having to meet a criterion for statistical significance. Often in a study the appearance of a few adverse events will be enough to provide a signal that there is a risk with a given therapy, though the numbers of adverse events are few and don't meet the criteria for statistical significance. The accepted approach is to err on the side of caution and assume the adverse event is not occurring by chance. This bias may incriminate a drug or therapeutic approach unfairly. The infrequency of adverse events in studies with trials being underpowered to reveal adverse events has the consequence that exposure to hundreds of patients may not reveal an uncommon side effect. In pharmaceutical studies exposure of a drug to several thousand patients may be inadequate to reveal hepatic toxicity of a drug that occurs in one and a thousand patients. Some are surprised that the average size drug development program does not reveal all infrequent but serious side effects. The occurrence of side effects post drug approval with a far greater patient exposure is not uncommon or the fault of drug developers or regulators. Adverse events should be evaluated in a study based on an "on treatment analysis". Events that occur in patients not administered the treatment or the alternative therapy are not events connected to the treatment although they could be related to study procedures such as withholding medications or treatments.

Assessment of Adverse Effects

There are a number of ways to obtain information during a trial as to the occurrence of adverse effects (AE). One can wait for an AE to be volunteered by a study subject. This avoids biasing the situation by suggesting the possibility of a given adverse event. But patients may often fail to report AE's, even ones that a physician might consider serious. One can during a study administer at pre-assigned times a systematic questionnaire(s) asking if the subject experienced a side effect. Sometimes a systematic review of systems can be employed. This is very thorough but invariably elicits long lists of complaints that would not otherwise be volunteered by the subject. One can alternatively ask directed questions relating to a specific side effect or system. This tends to increase the volunteering of symptoms that may be suggested by the question. Though a directed question ensures that a potential AE is not missed and that patients are focused on an area of interest. A problem is that this type of directed questioning may illicit minor or imaginary symptoms. There is no best way to survey for side effects in a study. It depends on the need to ensure that an area is covered by questioning and the importance of reporting infrequent, minor symptoms that would be otherwise overlooked by study participants. For the pharmaceutical developer or the advocate of a therapeutic approach, a direct question or system review requires a blinded study with a control group to ensure that unrelated or questioning suggested AE's are being obtained at no greater frequency in the treatment group as in the control group. Having a control gives a mechanism to establish baseline frequency of AE's. Consent forms that specifically mention a potential adverse event increases the reporting of these AE's, necessitating an appropriate control group to be able to attribute or not the AE to the intervention. Failing to have a control group in these situations will lead to many complaints considered as intervention related side effects when they may not be.

When assessing the reliability AE's and their relation to the intervention the frequency of their occurrence and the occurrence in separate patients increases the reliability of the reports. The longer the trial lasts the more likely to have AE's reported, especially those of low frequency or those that take time to develop. This is one of the most important reasons that a trial should have a duration that is as long as the clinical treatment period proposed for the agent. If the treatment is for years, then the initial exposure should be at least for one year. Follow up is needed for even a longer period than just the exposure, since the consequences of treatment in terms of AE development may not be seen for a period of time following exposure. An example was the higher incidence of MI's in patients treated with the NSAID Viox (Rofecoxib) where the increased frequency in MI's were only seen months after the treatment was stopped. A delayed signal of risk needs to be considered when one is designing the patient follow up period in a trial. The duration of exposure and the intensity of exposure may also be critical. There could be a threshold period being requisite for the development of the AE. Medications that are to be taken for years poses difficult issues as to trial duration. Exposure for a few months cannot reveal the possibility of adversity several years later. However, one can't study a drug for 5 or 10 years before approval. Usually for medications that will be taken for decades at least a year of exposure is advisable with longer post marketing surveillance.

Individual Susceptibility to an AE

An adverse event occurring in all patients suggests a dose is being employed at a toxic level. Few AE's occur in all patients, suggesting that most AE's are due to the unique genetic makeup of the individual. When assessing an AE, one needs to take into account the age, gender, disease state and genetics of the patient(s) who manifests the AE. The stage of the disease, genetic profile of the subject and the dose of the drug may all relate to the possibility of an AE occurring. One needs to consider concomitant therapy. The toxicity may be related to a drug-drug additive effect on a receptor, as for instance bradycardia due to the combined use of a beta blocker and a calcium channel blocker of the verapamil or diltiazem type. An AE may be due to a drug-drug interaction such that one drug blocks the metabolism of a second agent causing toxicity due to an excess amount of the drug building up due in poor metabolizes. An example of this is the cimetidine lidocaine interaction where cimetidine blocks lidocaine's metabolism causing excessive lidocaine levels that can lead to seizure, somnolence and coma. Besides drug interactions, one can observe an AE in some patients at lower doses than would otherwise be seen. This enhanced sensitivity may be due to poor metabolism due to a genetic enzymatic insufficiency, an increase absorption of a standard dose, or a decrease in a drug's elimination. All these possibilities need to be explored when evaluating an AE.

Reporting Adverse Events

When reporting an adverse event, a good description of the AE is important. One should estimate the severity and obtain the patient's estimation as well. Did the AE cause the subject to stop participating in the study? Did the AE cause a hospitalization, death or a permanent disability? What was the frequency of the AE re-occurring if the treatment continued? If treatment was stopped, what was the duration of the AE? Did it result in a lasting adversity? What was the temporal association between starting therapy and the AE developing?

AE's often don't involve the patient stopping therapy. The duration of the AE should be noted as the therapy was continued. If the frequency of treatment was reduced did the AE subside? If the patient stopped treatment and the AE subsided and then re-started when the study treatment began again that would be strong evidence that the AE was treatment related. If the investigator deliberately re-challenges the patient with a treatment to determine the likelihood of an association of the therapy with the AE, that goes beyond the study and should be considered a re-challenge investigation that should have IRB and patient approval with consent obtained.

The method of analysis of a trial may influence the frequency of AE reporting. If a trial is only analyzed by an intent to treat methodology, then patients who stop therapy, drop out or were lost to follow up will not report AE's and then the presence of an AE and its frequency will be lost. On treatment analysis is a more conservative approach to ascertain AE's. Counting the patients actually taking the therapy ensures that the AE's will be observed, and the AE's true incidence determined. However, it should be understood that an AE may be the reason for patient discontinuation, "lost to follow up". If at all possible, these considerations need to be excluded as possible outcomes due to an AE.

Reporting an AE should include:

Description of event

Frequency

Time from exposure to event

Dose level of therapy

Persistence or duration of the AE

Percentage of participants who permanently discontinued therapy due to AE

Estimation of the relation of AE to treatment (strongly associated, associated, possibly associated, unlikely and not associated)

Reducing AE Occurrences

Depending on how a trial is designed, the frequency of AE's can be increase or diminished by design. Healthier patients often have fewer AE's. By adjusting the inclusion and exclusion criteria of a study one can reduce the severity of disease, reduce the number of concomitant disease and thus enroll healthier patients less likely to have adverse events. By limiting concomitant medications, OTC products, herbal remedies, one can reduce the possibility of a drug interaction or the altering of drug metabolism and thus reduce AE incidence. The reduced follow up of a study also reduces the period for AE's to develop. It turns out that patients entering studies or study volunteers, tend to have less side effects. Thus, it is not uncommon to have more AE's reported in patients outside of studies than those in clinical trials. The generalizability of clinical trial AE reporting to the population at large may be limited with the possibility of unexpected AE's and more frequent AE's in the general population.

Adverse Drug Reactions with Pharmaceutical Products

Adverse event reporting with pharmaceutical products in

clinical drug development entails statutory requirements. An adverse event that may or may not be due to the agent under study must be reported to the sponsor of the study and the IRB. If there is no sponsor involved, the investigator must report to the FDA. The sponsor or investigator must report to the FDA any serious adverse drug reaction (ADR). An adverse drug reaction can be considered one that leads to a hospitalization, or prolongs a hospitalization, any occurrence that leads to a serious disability, or death must be reported. An adverse reaction that causes a congenital defect also must be reported. An adverse reaction that was unexpected, that is not noted in the Investigator Brochure, must be reported. The association of the drug to the event should be evaluated as remotely possible, possible, probable, or definite. These assessments are difficult and the difference between possible and probable is subjective. A definite assessment requires a re-challenge. This re-challenge requires consenting of the patient with IRB approved protocol for the purpose of the re-challenge. This is different than a pause in administration and resumption of the therapy that then may lead to the recurrence of the AE. Pausing therapy for a short period, or dose reduction is common practice and differs from a re-challenge study. The resumption of therapy when a serious side effect is suspected may not be advisable.

There are timelines for reporting. Serious ADR should be reported with a notification within 7 days to FDA with a follow up report within 15 days. Nonserious, expected ADR can be included in the annual report along with all study non-related, hospitalization and deaths reported with the disease state being studied.

Subsequent to a new drug approval, quarterly reports for 3 years and then annually are required.

Characterization of Adverse Events and Adverse Drug Reactions

Adverse events are untoward medical occurrences associated with the use of a drug in man whether or not considered drug related. An adverse drug reaction may not be considered an adverse event if the occurrence of the event is expected and unrelated to the study medication. Death and all adverse life-threatening events should be reported to FDA. An event is "life-threatening" if in the view of the investigator or sponsor, its occurrence places the patient or subject at immediate risk of death. Serious adverse events are serious if in the view of the investigator or sponsor can result in death, or a life-threatening event, hospitalization, prolongation of hospitalization, development of a persistent or significant incapacity, or substantial disruption of the ability to conduct normal life function, or the development of a congenital abnormality, or a birth defect. A suspected adverse reaction means any adverse event for which there is a reasonable possibility that a drug caused the adverse event. For the purpose of IND safety reporting, reasonable means there is evidence to suggest a causal relationship between the drug and the adverse event. A suspected adverse reaction implies to FDA a lesser degree of certainty about causality than adverse reaction which means any adverse event probably caused by a drug. An unexpected adverse event or unexpected adverse reaction is considered unexpected if the occurrence is not listed in the drug's current Investigator Brochure, or its severity is greater than that described in the Investigator Brochure. An IND safety report in writing should be reported to FDA as soon as possible, but at least within 15 days of the occurrence. All participating investigators in a multi-center study should also be notified. All serious and unexpected, adverse reactions must be reported. The IND safety report is submitted in narrative format using FDA form 3500A, or in an electronic format. If the event is unexpected, fatal, or life-threatening it must be reported as soon as possible, but no later than 7 calendar days after the sponsor's initial receipt of the information followed up by a more extensive written report in 15 days.

Reporting study endpoints such as mortality or major morbidity – hospitalization in an IND safety report is not required unless there is evidence suggesting a causal relationship between the drug and the event. If there is a suspected causal relationship, then the death or morbidity must be reported even if it is a study endpoint. If the event is a study endpoint and not suspected as drug related the event is reported in the annual IND report.

In a study on the efficacy of IV amiodarone in cardiac arrest patients the FDA instructed the principal investigator to report all deaths in an annual report and not as individual safety reports because death was expected for most cardiac arrest patients, and it was unlikely the deaths in the study were associated with the treatment with amiodarone. The mortality was high in the study, at 24 hours 56% were dead on amiodarone and 90% of those receiving lidocaine, the standard therapy at that time. While amiodarone increased survival, mortality was high and in both groups unlikely to be related to the drug administered.

Pharmacovigilance

There is a field dedicated to the enumeration and assessment of adverse events. Pharmacovigilance is not limited to assessment of adverse events during a clinical trial, but adversity from a therapeutic agent in the course of its utilization in any situation, pre or post approval. There are a number of databases that compile AE's that can be very useful for those assessing an agent, as well as those interested in research in this area. The FDA adverse event reporting system called FAERS is one such database. The material is provided by pharmaceutical companies as part of their mandatory reporting as well as information provided by physicians, and patients on a voluntary basis. There is the possibility of double reporting of an AE, but most experts believe FAERS undercounts AEs with limited physician and patient reporting. Sentinel events are AEs reported by hospitals as classified by the Joint Commission and are also included in the FAERS database. Those interested in studying AE's and their reporting system will find the FAERS reporting system a useful source of information. Unfortunately, the FAERS system is unreliable to determine the frequency of an AE Since many AE's are not reported. The frequency of an AE found in FAERS should be considered the minimal incidence. Of course all reports may not be AE's but a happenstance association.

Chapter 14
The Trial in Operation

Once the trial is designed, funded, approved by the IRB and the study case report forms are created the investigator needs to proceed to patient screening. It is useful to keep a recruitment log to identify patients that were screened. Those patients not entering the study may possibly be recycled if the situation warrants. Baseline measurements need to be collected as the study progresses to be able to assess the comparability of the groups to see if imbalances have been avoided, imbalances that can affect study results. If imbalances are identified this may require stratification of the data when it comes time for analysis.

Data Collection

The collection of data is a key component of the study. A thoughtful, workable plan for continuous data collection, including the patient characteristics, study endpoints, adverse events, and study adherence are essential. Without a well-planned data collection program critical information can be missed, lost or may require a difficult post study attempt at retrieval that may be arduous and time consuming. Post study data retrieved is fraught with inaccuracy and bias and should not be needed if a study's data collection procedures are well planned in advance.

Data to Collect

Baseline information

Primary response variable results

Secondary response variable(s) results

Adverse outcomes, adverse events

Study adherence

The data collection process should aim to collect all the demographic and initial patient information collected on participants at baseline, at each study visit (real or virtual) including all contacts the subject makes with the study staff. However, the investigator must avoid the "nice to know" trap in data collection. In many studies too much inconsequential data, tangential to the study is often collected. Large studies employ a data collection staff and a dedicated coordinator(s) who has the capacity to handle a large, unwieldy data base. However, even in large studies too much data can lead to excessive time and cost expended and can lead to critical information and safety signals being missed. Small investigator driven studies can be adversely impacted with excessive data collection, jeopardizing the study.

Problems with data can consist of missing data, incorrect data, or poor quality data. Poor data quality may be due to poor measurement techniques causing excessive variability. These problems can lead to delays in study analysis and reporting or at worst inaccurate results and a failed study. Missing data can severely question a study's reliability. Every effort on the part of study monitors needs to be made to obtain missing data. If a patient misses a visit, the study visit needs to be re-scheduled or the data obtained at a follow up visit. To avoid incorrect data the data collection process should have procedures imbedded such as a review of the recorded data by a second study coordinator or possible the use of "double entry" technique for data entry and tabulation where the data is entered twice and only data that matches from both entrees is collected. Data that is rejected needs to be checked and reentered for the data to be counted. The standardization of measurement techniques, the use of trained personnel for the administration of questions minimizing differences in a surveys administration can go a long way to diminish variability. Laboratory values and clinical laboratory data ranges needs to be standardized and outlies in the data re-checked before entry.

Minimizing Poor Data

The case report form that is employed to collect data needs to be carefully planned and the forms utility periodically reviewed during the study. Data that is the result of interpretation needs to have the interpretation variables defined in the study manual. Normal ranges in laboratory data need to be provided if data comes from individual sites as opposed to a central core laboratory. Laboratory data must have a standardized normal range for the data entered. If data is collected by staff interviews the questions must be standardized and the manner the questions are asked be as consistent as possible. Even experienced staff needs training in the questioning technique to maintain a standardized approach. Staff training is needed at all levels. All staff needs general training in ethics and informed consent. CITI or NIH training with certification is needed for staff. Beyond the basic training there is trial specific training that is needed for the clinical staff as well as the study research assistants who are usually the ones tasked with data collection. If clinical events need to be adjudicated this needs to be done by clinical observers who consistently adjudicate all events and the observers need to be blinded as to study intervention to avoid bias.

Mechanisms of Data Collection

When I first became involved in clinical studies in the 1970's, data was collected on paper in study workbooks and then tabulated. If the events were part of a multi-center study the site data would be collected by monitors and then re-entered into tables at as central site. This process was fraught with the potential for inaccurate entries and misinterpretation. Hand collection of data may still take place at a small single site study, often investigator sponsored studies. However, the information age has greatly changed the data collection process. Most studies have electronic case report forms, often they are interactive, questioning entries that are outside an expected range. The data is shared with a central data collection entity of the study, often simultaneously. The accuracy of such systems are excellent and facilitate rapid recognition of the need to re-check data entry or if data is missing, the need for it to be obtained and then entered. Still, data entry mistakes are possible, missing data may not be obtained and thus appropriate data collection monitoring is still needed.

Monitoring

To ensure the quality of the study data monitoring is critical. Monitoring should start early. Either with internal study site monitoring or external monitoring. The first collection of data should be monitored early to ensure optimum reliability of data which can substantially increase the quality of the study. A schedule should be set for repeated and periodic monitoring. A good monitoring program needs to take into consideration feedback from those being monitored and adjustment of data collection procedures when necessary. Monitoring can be done on a selective basis reviewing a random sample or each and every case can be reviewed. The more frequent and more extensive the monitoring the more reliable the data. Monitoring does consume a substantial amount of time and this must be taken into consideration. A more intensive monitoring program needs to allow for increased staff and the costs entailed. In a multi-center study, a site that has persistent problems with data record keeping needs more training or if the problem is not able to be resolved dropped from the trial.

Study audits are a form of monitoring. They may be scheduled or at times initiated with little notice. Studies under FDA supervision may be subject to an FDA audit. Often these audits are for cause due to a complaint by a participant, study personnel, or a sponsor. Studies that contribute a substantial number of patients or participate in a pivotal study can expect to be monitored. Sponsors may audit a study in addition to monitoring on a routine or on a random basis. Audits of sites with data discrepancies are more likely to be unscheduled.

Patient Adherence

As a trial progresses it is important that the investigator track patient adherence to the study protocol. Patients failing to keep appointments who miss assigned lab test, or fail to comply with scheduled medical procedures or testing can be a serious problem for the study. It is important to identify these problems early on and correct the problem, trying to improve compliance. In the design of a study thought should be given to procedures that identify non-compliance. Missing an appointment or a lab test should be immediately flagged and the appointment or test rescheduled. Patients failing to reschedule need to be contacted early and repeatedly. It is important to maintain communication with patients. Most patients have cell phones and the phones can be utilized to send reminders for follow up and fulfilling scheduled appointments. Text messages to patients and if need be, contacting family member to contact and remind patients can also be considered.

There are usually patients who have compliance issues. It is good to try and identify these patients before they are included in the study. Unfortunately, some patients show such poor compliance that they may need to be dropped from the study. Some subjects just cease contacting the study staff and are lost to follow up. Patients have a right to withdraw from a study and can't and should not be forced to comply. In these cases, a patient study "drop out" should be asked for a reason and this should be recorded in the patient's record. That a patient is lost to follow up should be noted in the patient's record. A lost to follow up patient can severely impact a study. Too large a number of lost to follow up patients can distort study outcomes and compromise study results. While the investigator can't guarantee that patients will comply or not be lost to follow up, investigators can insert in the consent that all data till the patient withdraws that has been collected will be used in the study reports. Additionally, all consents should include a statement that patients lost to follow up can be traced as to outcome by the investigator reviewing hospital records, reviewing death registries such as the one run by the Social Security Administration and by contacting the patient at a later date for follow up. Obtaining this information if it is agreed to in the initial consent is permitted and appropriate.

Many patients miss appointments due to weather and transportation issues. It is advisable that studies provide for easy rescheduling of appointments, laboratory tests and procedures and that the study provides assistance with transportation. Operating in Chicago, as I have done for years, requires ingenuity. Not enrolling patients in studies with frequent follow up in the worst winter months and providing transportation when weather creates obstacle to patient adherence can greatly aid patients in conforming to the study schedule.

Keeping patients informed as to study progress, the purpose of the study, and how the subjects are contributing to medical science and public health can go a long way in enhancing patient compliance. Creating a study newsletter for large studies can enhance patient and staff interest and improve study adherence. It is useful to keep patients informed as to study progress creating a sense that the patient is part of the study team and making an important contribution to the study. A study is usually focused on a particular health issue while patients need to maintain medical care in other areas independent of the study. It is important for the study staff to be attentive to other medical needs of the study participants providing advice and assistance. This furthers the development of a bond between study personnel and patients and helps ensure the continued participation and compliance by patients.

In pharmaceutical studies one usually wants to evaluate study medication compliance. The evaluation of compliance can be as simple as asking the patient if they have taken their medication. Pill counts of returned medication may be helpful, but patients could dispose of unused pills. One can undertake toxicology studies evaluating urine content for drug or its metabolite(s), or the blood levels of the therapeutic agent. In the last few years surveillance techniques have become more complex with pill containers reporting on the opening of the container and the time opened to see if patients are compliant. However, even here the pill could have been removed from the container at the correct time, but not taken. To counter this possibility the medication can be tracked with a signal that permits determination that the pill was actually swallowed by the patient. These can be very intrusive procedures and are only recommended in very special circumstances. Urine sampling is far easier and a reliable method when drug compliance needs monitoring. When there are physiologic manifestations of drug compliance they can be used effectively. Drugs that slow heart rate can be assessed for patient compliance with a simple measurement of heart rate. The report of certain consistent side effects may correlate with compliance.

Monitoring Patient Response Outcomes

It is important to monitor the study to determine if the study procedure and data collection are proceeding without problems. But it's also important to monitor the study outcomes. Is the primary study endpoint occurring at a required frequency to be able to accept or reject the null hypothesis? Are there adverse trends developing or adverse side effects being observed that question the continuance of a study? These are difficult but important questions. Difficult because the study is most often blinded, and the investigators will not know if the adverse outcome or adverse drug reactions are due to the intervention or occurring in the no treatment or placebo arm of the study. In a single center study often, the investigator may monitor outcomes blinded. If a concerning trend develops the question arises if the study should be paused or stopped. If the investigator unblinds the study, then future data obtained may be biased. Thus, a mechanism is needed for a person or committee independent from the study to evaluate the outcomes and determine how to proceed. In a small or single center study the trends can be evaluated in a blinded fashion and if adversity is suspected, or the trend crosses a pre-specified boundry then a third party can be consulted to evaluate the study, unblinding the study to advise on the advisability of proceeding. A study can have a non-study investigator serve as a safety officer (SO) who can review data in a blinded (or unblinded) fashion looking for signals alerting to adversity or data collection problems. Even in small or single center studies most IRB's are now requiring a data safety monitoring plan where boundaries for stopping and procedures for outcome evaluation are specified in advance. Pre-specifying boundaries for pausing or stopping the study are critical. Without pre-specifying boundaries, a trial may so unnerve a monitor or committee as to cause the study to be prematurely stopped, ending the ability of the study to answer the question the study was designed to resolve. However, the stopping boundary needs to take into consideration that the patients in the study need to be protected from harm. Once the potential risks of the study have substantially changed it would be unethical to proceed in order to definitively determine a study outcome. Another problem that arises is that multiple statistical evaluations of a study endpoint can reduce power of the study and can thus increase the possibility that the study misses a positive outcome resulting in a false negative result. Repeated testing can be a serious problem and thus performing repeated statistical analysis must be kept to a minimum and the initial statical assumptions such as study power and sample size need to allow for the possibility of repeated testing by increasing sample size. There are statistical techniques that can adjust statistical requirements for significance, allowing for multiple testing.

The Data Safety Monitoring Board (DSMB)

The data safety monitoring board or committee (DSMB) has been created to provide monitoring of a blinded study such that individuals familiar with the study procedures and statistical issues can follow outcome trends and adverse event trends as they unfold during a study. For observational studies with vulnerable populations there may be created an Observational Data Safety Monitoring Board (ODSMB). The committee is usually constituted before a study starts and creates scheduled times to evaluate study trends established in advance. The DSMB usually has a statistician to assist in their evaluation of trends. The DSMB is charged with difficult responsibilities. The DSMB must look out for the patient's safety and not permit a trial to continue if it will lead to a significant number of adverse outcomes. What is a significant number and are the trends real or occurring by happenstance is the committee conundrum. If a study is stopped permanently, all the efforts, the resources provided to the study can be lost and the question the study is attempting to resolve may go unanswered. If the study continues and harms accumulate when the study should have been stopped that can be most unfortunate. Thus, a DSMB needs to make difficult decisions in an unbiased manner while protecting patients. There is the issue of a study continuing beyond the point needed to obtain statistically significant data that rejects the null hypothesis. Continuing a study that has clear results rejecting the null hypothesis is wrong, but prematurely stopping a study for what is initially thought of as an early success has sometimes led to a premature termination with the primary hypothesis questioned when the study is reported. A study may also be terminated for futility when there is little to no chance that the study will have a positive outcome. The DSMB may also suggest that participant participation or entry of new patients needs to be extended such that the event rate is increased to increase the probability of success of the study. Besides continued enrollment another strategy to improve the chances of success is for the study to be extended to permit more events to occur. Studies may also be extended for longer observation periods to observe for adverse events.

How the DSMB makes the evaluation can be critical. The DSMB can be un blinded as to intervention or control groups, or the DSMB can be blinded as are the investigators and study personnel making the study triple blinded (patients, investigators, and the DSMB blinded). Having served on a number of DSMB's I can say that being blinded makes decision making far more difficult, dramatically prolonging deliberation. However, not knowing which group is treated and which is not, removes a great potential for bias. If adversity trends in the intervention group, it is human nature to be cautious and often a study is stopped prematurely. If the DSMB is blinded, then equipoise is more likely and the DSMB is more likely to require a more substantial signal of harm to prematurely stop a study. It clearly is in the sponsor's interest to have a blinded DSMB as well as in the interest of science. Bringing studies to fruition, answering an important issues in clinical medicine is a high priority as is the prevention of harm to patients.

The evaluation of events is made easier if the time from exposure to treatment and the development of adversity is short. When there is a long latent period between treatment and an adverse event, determination of an association is more difficult and a decision to discontinue a study by the DSMB is made more difficult.

The issue of multiple testing and the "spending of alpha" is not a trivial issue. If a DSMB evaluates the primary outcome variable five times and the initial alpha was at 0.05 the chance of a false positive being reached increases from 5% to 15 to 20%. The analysis can be adjusted statistically such that a greater difference between intervention and control can be required to obtain statistical significance. To compensate for the multiple testing one can employ the simplest correction formula, Bonferoni, where the correction is α/k, where K is the number of tests resulting in the new α required. If the α is <0.05 and undertaking 5 tests the new α would be 0.01 to reach a comparable significant outcome as if alpha was tested once. In deciding on the number of statistical tests that will be performed during the course of the study one must consider that as alpha is spent the number of participating subjects may need to be increased. If the trial is ongoing and the event rate is not as predicted the requirement for conditional power or the probability that the test statistic will be greater than the critical value chosen for significance decreases and the study enrollment needs to be increased. As the study progresses, if events are such as to be greater than predicted the conditional power has increased while if the events are less than predicted, conditional power has decreased. This type of evaluation may be very helpful in making a decision to extend or shorten the duration of a study.

Data Safety Monitoring Plan Outline

A data safety monitoring plan can be drafted with the following sections:

Description of study design

Description of study management

Participant safety

Potential risks

Potential benefits

Informed consent process

Reportable events and procedures for reporting

Interim analysis and stopping rules

Data safety monitoring procedures

Data management

Data Security

Quality control

Quality assurance

Of late, IRB's are requiring a Data Safety Monitoring Plan for all clinical trials; small single center, or large multi-center studies

Chapter 15

Closing a Study and Data Analysis

When the study has been completed a number of steps must be undertaken to properly complete the study and analyze the data. Completion of a study can occur when the planned evaluation is complete, when the time to conduct the study has expired and will not be extended, when finances have been depleted, or a decision has been made to stop the study. The stopping decision can be because the study has clearly shown a positive outcome for the primary response variable. The study could be stopped for futility, no hope of rejecting the null hypothesis, or the study could be stopped due to adversity, an unacceptable number of adverse drug reactions, or procedural adversities have been reported. Another reason for stopping may be that the sponsor may have withdrawn the drug or device from further testing. Whatever the reason for stopping, the study needs to be closed in an orderly fashion with all extent data collected. The data needs to be analyzed and reported. If a trial is negative, stopped for futility, or stopped for adversity, the results are important to report. Publication of the trial results may avoid another group of researchers pursuing the same or similar research question.

The Study Closeout

There are a number of ways to end a study. The study could be stopped all at once. This can be a tremendous burden to investigators and staff. If a study site is following a hundred patients and all are stopped at once and each patient needs a 1-hour final visit that can take a month to schedule and see all the patients, a full-time enterprise. Unfortunately, due to an abrupt stopping of a study the "all at once closeout" is sometimes forced upon investigators. The preferred approach would be a closeout usually based on "time in time out" approach. A pre-specified time for follow up is prescribed in the protocol. As each patient reaches the time allotted, they complete their participation in the study. Since enrollment is stopped as patients are assessed into the study, so is the completion of patients staggered.

The last visit should not be considered the study closeout. The last visit is a data collection point, while the closeout visit may still collect data it also functions as the time for a number of operational considerations to be completed. Equipment lent to the patient may be collected. Medications that are unused will be collected and accounted for. The patient's therapy may be unblinded and communicated to the participant. This may be a complicated decision if the termination process is staggered, since patients unblinded may share information with staff and fellow patients in the study, effectively unblinding the study for other patients prematurely. Sometimes knowing what medication the patient was on is important to base recommendations for subsequent therapy. If this is the case, then the unblinding process can be assigned to a single physician who uses the knowledge of medication assignment to prescribe follow-up therapy. This can be a complicated process and thus many studies only unblind when all patients have completed the study. The unblinding process should not extend to the staff who will analyze the results. Otherwise, the study will be analyzed unblinded and then for all intense and purpose the study might not be considered an a blinded study.

Follow-up treatment needs to be recommended for patients. For therapies that may cause a rebound effect when stopped, the patients may need to be gradually withdrawn at the time of the last visit with the withdrawal extending to the time of the closeout visit. As a medical student, I worked on the first propranolol angina study and had the unfortunate experience of seeing two study patients who were doing well on maximal propranolol therapy, stop treatment and have a myocardial infarction within 24 hours. At that time the consequences of sudden withdrawal of beta blockers were not understood and the concept of rebound formative. Today researchers need to be aware of the risks of stopping a treatment suddenly to avoid adverse outcomes.

The closeout visit may be a point in the patient's treatment where no further intervention is provided, but there may be interest in continued patient surveillance. If this is done for the safety of the patient this is appropriate medical therapy. However, if this becomes a research project, a protocol should be developed with IRB approval obtained and consent from the patient. Many studies have a codicil that provides for continued follow-up for months or years to collect safety information. A study may come to an end but offer patients who have benefited from a treatment to continue therapy. This may be termed an "open-label" study. An open label study can benefit the patient, and also used to collect long-term safety information. Such a study needs to be in the protocol and consent form, or a new follow up study initiated with consent obtained.

Data Retrieval

Every effort needs to be made to minimize "lost to follow-up" patients. The closeout visit can be an opportunity to try and make contact with "lost to follow-up" patients, attempting to obtain follow up data. Patients with missing data can have the problem corrected at the close out visit, or at least an explanation for the missing appointment, test, or procedure entered into the case report form. It is important to resolve issues with data as soon as possible, while the patient has a recollection of what happened, and you have the patient in front of you to question. While some studies have virtual closeouts, it is best to have the last visit as a face-to-face meeting with the patient to resolve information issues, obtain feedback and provide future guidance to the patient. During a study the investigator and staff often become the primary physician on many health matters. Patients referred need to be re-referred to their referring physician and those who may have been recruited by advertising recommended for follow-up to physicians willing to take on new patients.

Storage of Study Supplies and Data

Medications are usually returned to the sponsor, or at the sponsor's instructions destroyed at the study site. A careful record of these returns or destruction needs to be kept. Study records should be safely stored, and a copy stored separately. In this day and age of electronic storage appropriate data protection is essential. Backup storage is important to secure. Data on a computer hard drive needs to be backed up on a memory stick, CD, in the cloud or other reliable secondary storage sites so it can't be lost or degraded. Storage in a remote site, "the cloud" can be an appropriate backup. Back up is essential to safeguard data collected after years of work collecting the data and having patients take part in a study that may offer risk. Laboratory data, graphics (x-ray, Echos, CT scans, angiograms, etc.) need to be stored. These materials may have been re-interpreted at a core laboratory for consistency of results. The material needs to be stored at the study site and the core laboratory with their final interpretation. Depending on clinical data storage at a hospital or medical practice may make secondary review more difficult. Clinical sites can purge certain clinical data and may not store information as long as investigators may have a need to review the material. I once was interested in the 24-hour tape recording of ECGs (Holter's) from a landmark study for analysis to determine if there was a predictive ECG marker for risk. However, after tracking down the Holter tapes from a number of studies they were either lost, stored at conditions that made the re-analysis impossible, or were so incomplete as to identifiers that made them useless. Planning for future utilization requires reliable storage. The costs of storage should be considered in planning potential landmark studies. Data storage costs over many years can be expensive.

Planning the Study Closeout

There are costs involved at all stages of a study and the closeout has to be planned and has costs that must be covered. Employee allocation needs to be considered. The place, type and cost of data storage and ensuring security for patient confidentiality needs to be planned. Optimizing data collection, storage and data curation needs to be planned and executed during the study and provided for through the study closeout. For the investigator supported by a sponsor, the study closeout is the time to arrange for final payment including future data storage costs. Advanced planning is advisable. At the time of the site closeout all accounts should be settled with the sponsor.

Reporting Results

Patients in the study need to be informed of the study results. Due to blinding considerations that may not occur at the study closeout. But informing the patient should be done as soon as possible. Waiting years is unsatisfactory to patients. Referring physicians and those physicians who will follow up with the patient should also be informed. Colleagues who have assisted in carrying out the study, those that referred patients and supported the study should also be informed. There are contractual and legal reporting responsibilities. The IRB needs to receive a report on the study at its completion. If the study is supported by an NIH grant, there are specific reporting requirements to the NIH that need to be completed. Sponsors from the pharmaceutical or medical device companies that are supporting the study need a report on the study's outcome. Pharmaceutical or Medical Device companies are responsible for reporting study results to FDA. Society sponsors such as the American Cancer Society, or the American Heart Association require a final study report.

Most clinical trials are registered usually with ClinicalTrials.gov. A report to these registration entities is required at the completion of the study. At the appropriate time investigators may want to report findings to the public, usually with the help of an institutional press office, press release or press conference. This is best done in conjunction with an institution's public relations office. Any public release of information needs to be coordinated with the sponsor and if a multi-centered study is involved coordination with the management of the study should be done. It is inappropriate for a single site to release information on a multi-site study. A press release, or publications are to be made through a central coordinating committee. It is important that investigators or study participants should not learn of the study results through the press. The study participants have taken part in a study, provided personal information, agreed to take part despite potential risks and thus should receive the study results directly from the investigator or his associates.

Studies that have found results that may contribute to clinical practice may also see result information disseminated through the National Library of Medicine, or through "Dear Doctor letter" by the FDA. These communications through FDA, NIH, or NCI most often are outside the control of the investigators.

Reporting results also needs to be coordinated with any intellectual property constraints. Premature disclosure before patent protection may establish prior art that precludes a patent. This can be an economic disaster for a sponsor but can also limit the potential benefit of a therapy. A product without intellectual property protection may not be developed further or marketed because the reduced potential for compensation may severely limit the product's earning potential.

Study Analysis

The analysis of study results can at times be rather straightforward. The statistical methods for analysis should have been stated in the protocol, the critical statistical methods for analysis of the primary and secondary endpoints should have been pre-specified and the data points and methods of reporting (intention to treat or on treatment analysis) pre-specified. However, in the course of the analysis of results many questions can arise that may not have been anticipated.

Intent to Treat Analysis or On Treatment Analysis

What patients should be analyzed is an often-disputed point. Which patients to analyze should have been determined when the study was initially planned. The "gold standard" of analysis "intention to treat" means any subject randomized should be considered in the analysis. This approach removes bias and is the most rigorous approach. A study analyzed by the intention to treat principle that is found to be significant has met a high standard. However, I would contend that on treatment analysis may often be more informative for clinicians. One wants to know if those who took the treatment are indeed benefited. One can criticize on treatment analysis for not accounting for problems with the therapy that leads to non-compliance. However, the adverse event profile will give an indication of the toxicities, as does the treatment arm's dropout rate. It is best to report results both in terms of on treatment and intention to treat analysis. The intention to treat analysis will reveal if the therapy is effective and if patients comply with therapy. An excellent example of this issue is a study with amiodarone in heart failure. With an on-treatment analysis the drug reduced sudden death, but with an intention to treat analysis amiodarone failed to show benefit. This is because a large number of patients stopped amiodarone therapy because it was poorly tolerated which led to many in the intention to treat group not receiving drug and thus in all probability continued to have arrhythmias that lead to death.

Protocol Eligibility

Another issue is protocol eligibility. Patients can be entered into a protocol that do to meet study inclusion or exclusion criteria. Some patients may not have the disease being studied by mistake, incorrect diagnostic lab test, or deliberate action by investigators. Should these patients be excluded from study analysis? Excluding ineligible patients by the investigator has too much potential for bias. It is best for a study to have a careful screening process and for the patients that enter the study ensuring that only eligible patients are entered. If ineligible patients are still entered and can be identified the study should be analyzed with and without these patients. Some studies enter patients into the study before a definitive diagnosis can be made. Conditions such as an acute myocardial infarction or stroke may only be definitively determined hours after a patient is entered into the study. What first may seem to be an MI, alternatively could be an acute coronary syndrome (ACS). Instead of a stroke it could be a transient ischemic attack (TIA). Even more problematic is that the therapy can abort the pathophysiology of a stroke converting the diagnosis to a TIA or acute coronary syndrome, short-circuiting the adverse outcome leaving only the prodrome. Probably the best approach is to analyze these studies on the basis of the initial diagnosis determined at randomization. One could also have an expert who is blinded to the therapy provided remove patients from analysis who turn out not to have the requisite diagnosis. By having a blinded assessor, one can reduce bias from affecting the analysis. Not excluding the patients who inappropriately entered the study can be problematic. However, excluding patients who have an event aborted by treatment may fail to show the true benefit of therapy. Whatever the analysis team decides it is best to fully describe the methods employed and the reason for patient exclusions.

Participant Adherence

Participants can fail to adhere to treatment. The degree of adherence can be estimated in advance and power of the study calculated on the basis of the estimation. Once again, the best approach is to analyze that data with and without the non-adherent patients. As part of a study analysis the investigator should perform an analysis for an interaction between study adherence and the intervention. Another. difficult issue is patients in a study who change arms of the study. Patients on one therapy may crossover to the alternative therapy often from the control to the intervention group. Patient receiving surgery may receive medical therapy or vice versa. A study comparing medical therapy of an acute appendicitis to surgical therapy may have a number of patients who crossover from the medical arm to the surgical arm. Some patients may receive antibiotics after surgery, the therapy in the medical treatment arm. Should these crossover patients be excluded? There is no definitive answer and once again, it is best to analyze and report the study results counting the crossovers and also reporting results leaving out those patients. Non- adherence reduces a studies power and that is why when making a sample size calculation consideration needs to be made to the possibility of "drop ins" and "dropouts". A study that finds a significant outcome when analyzed with and without compliant patients, as well as with and without crossovers presents much more robust results.

Missing or Corrupted Data

With data missing or poor quality one could take a simple approach and exclude the patients with data problems and proceed to study analysis. However, the reason for missing or poor data may be due to patient characteristic issues resulting from the arm of the study the patient is in and may factor into study outcome. Sicker patients may miss more appointments, older patients with reduced mobility show up for less visits or fewer prescribed tests. Study sites in areas with treacherous weather may see a higher incidence of missing data. A study intervention may cause more study visit compliance issues causing an imbalance of missing data in one arm of the study, biasing the study outcome.

There are methods to try and deal with data problems. Missing or non-intelligible data can be imputed. A crude but simple method is "last entry forward" where the previous entry is inserted again in the place of the missing entry. One can average the previous entries and then input a number for the missing entry. One can use a regression model to provide an entry. Another approach is to create multiple entries using a regression model and then analyze the data with multiple imputations. This can be the basis of a propensity score analysis where critical missing data is inputted with values at the extremes of the data range to see if outcome changes significantly with the different imputations. The consistency of the outcome with more extreme input supports the study's conclusion. However, if there is no previous entry or it is for a first occurrence of a study milestone, a natural history endpoint, such as hospitalization, intubation or death the imputation method may not be helpful.

Censoring missing data or unintelligible data can be an approach. If the missing data is infrequent, omitting the missing data point in the tabulation may be the approach with the least potential to introduce biases. However, studies with enough missing data to “tip” the result in a different direction is problematic.

Deciding which data to count is fraught with bias issues. The best approach is to minimize missing data as much as possible and if missing data is prevalent report the effects of the analysis that favor the null hypothesis. This is a conservative approach, safer than supporting a positive outcome on less than a robust data set.

Inconsistent Data

While I was a resident "moonlighting" in a cardiology laboratory, tabulating the results of an immunoassay for digoxin measurement, every so often I would come upon a number that was outrageously out of line with the majority of results, perhaps 10,000 times out of line. In laboratory work in the basic sciences, numbers that are so outrageous are for the most part attributed to an "accident" and are excluded. In pre-clinical work outliers are often dropped if the number is more than two standard deviations from the mean. While this leads to more consistent results, one needs to consider reasons for the outlier reading. As for digoxin, the results for years were attributed to "quenching" issue with the biologic sample regarding the lipid sintilation counter. It turned out years later the very high readings were due to endogenous digoxin-like substances found in some patients with heart failure. What is thought to be a "lab error" may turn out to be a very real phenomenon, even a major discovery.

It is easy to recommend that the results be reported with and without the outlier. But is this really feasible? I have not seen a paper with data presented including and excluding data outliers in a paper. The report would go on and on without anyone paying attention. The real problem of reporting outliers is that it can drastically increase variability which reduces power of the study. Best to omit outliers that are outside the pre-specified limits (perhaps 2 standard deviations). In an appendix to the study report what was done and the analysis results without any exclusions. This is most important if the exclusions affect the determination of statistical significance. In the age of publication addendums with online publishing that is easy to do and gives those with a need for reviewing results in depth, an opportunity to understand the full picture with all its blemishes, offering possible insights into unknown factors such as endogenous digoxin like substance.

Primary and Secondary Variables

Analysis of the primary and secondary endpoints follows the same considerations. Whether it be which participants to count, how non-compliance is handled, missing data, outlier results, competing events, covariate adjustments, multiple comparison, or the use of cut points, the handling of the primary and secondary endpoints are the same. Often in an analysis questions arise as to the different results obtained from subsets of the study population. These subsets or subgroups are best pre-specified and based on pre-identified characteristics. Subgroups that are created in the post study analysis period are subject to considerable biases since they are identified based on study outcomes. The more subgroups analyzed the greater the loss of study power due to multiple comparisons. One also has the problem of multiple comparisons leading to a positive finding due to chance, a Type I error (false positive). The subgroups should be based on characteristics of the study population that are thought to affect outcome. Subsets should have a biologic rationale for evaluation. Looking at outcomes in a heart failure population who had preserved as compared to reduced ejection fraction has a biologic rationale behind the selection of the subgroups. Evaluating similar subgroups that other studies have evaluated and finding similar results gives support to the selection of these subgroups and the associated findings. A subgroup that has a significant outcome when the overall results for the study population is negative must be treated as hypothesis generating and warrants confirmation in a future study. In a breast cancer study with Herceptin the women with Her-2 positive tumor receptors responded to Herceptin therapy. The conclusion was not that estrogen receptors negative, Her-2 positive tumor responded to Herceptin (a potential anti-tumor agent), but rather further study of this group would be needed to confirm efficacy of Herceptin in this subgroup of the breast cancer population.

Cut points

Another way to evaluate study outcome is to use the technique of creating cut points - divisions of the data set. This is usually employed in continuous data by dividing the continuous variable into groups. In hypertension studies one may divide the population into groups based on presenting BP, pre-hypertension with a BP systolic 129-139, mild hypertension (140-159), moderate (160-189) and severe hypertension systolic 190 or greater. This may be reasonable and if pre-specified is a sound basis for analysis.

Another approach is to review the data in tabular form and measured BP systolic and compare the BP level against outcome at 5 years. After reviewing the mortality data one may find an increase at a BP of 160 and higher associated with a higher mortality. The analysis would create group of BP 160 and below as one group and 161 and above as the second group. The cut point is specific to the data set and if one compares the two groups using a dichotomous statistical test one may very well determine statistical significance. This cut point is data driven and introduces a bias to the outcome of the study results that may indeed be accidental. Data driven cut points may be specific to a particular set of results and are a biased way to interpret data. Better to evaluate BP as a continuous variable and its association with risk.

Competing Events

In designing a study, one wants to capture the clinically significant events and determine if they show a difference that is statistically significance. However, if the patient in the study dies, goes to surgery, or has another disease altering event, that can drastically change all other study outcome measures that can bias the results. If patients in a study on the outcome of coronary angioplasty on survival dies the patient's subsequent occurrences can't be evaluated. If in the alternate treatment group more patients suffer MI's one may inappropriately conclude that the alternative treatment group causes more MI's, which would be false. This is one reason composite endpoints are often utilized especially when mortality is a likely outcome. Also, composite endpoints aggregate events, amplifying effect size and thus decreasing the required sample size to obtain at 80% power at an alpha of <0.05, for significance. The problem can arise that highly significant endpoints such as death can be comingled with much less clinically significant endpoints such as an enzyme elevation. In the angioplasty outcome example death is often comingled with MI occurrence and enzyme elevations. Cardiac enzyme elevations are of questionable significance (especially minor elevations). Counting enzyme release may yield a positive study result based on mostly enzyme differences between treated and untreated patients without the intervention affecting mortality. Using a composite endpoint including death and reporting a difference between groups gives the report more weight clinically than the outcome may actually deserve. Still composite endpoints can be helpful to avoid the problem of censoring events as well as to decrease sample size to more manageable numbers. However, there are limits to the benefits of using composite endpoints. Recently some investigators have tried to combine efficacy endpoints with a safety endpoint. With the evaluation of anti-thrombolytic agents or anti-platelet drugs some advocate combining death and the need for a repeat procedure with the adverse report of bleeding. The endpoints of efficacy and toxicity, (bleeding) may be competing, going in opposite directions and thus confuse the presentation of results. Clinically one wants to know the efficacy as well as the risk (bleeding) separately and then make a decision based on the risks versus the benefits. Combining benefit and risk in a single endpoint obscures the individual outcomes, especially in this instance when they may be moving in opposite directions.

Censoring Endpoints

In an analysis of a study, one may find a number of events early on. Can these events be censored because they occur in a period where the drug is unlikely to have had time to affect outcome? If the study has a pre-specified "blanking period" to exclude events because the time needed for a treatment effect has not occurred, one may exclude these events. Despite pre-specifying a blanking period, the potential for introducing bias is present. It may be that the treatment worsens the early outcome, and the treatment did have an effect, but it was adverse. By not counting the initial period one may bias the study creating a false positive outcome. IV ACE inhibitors given very early after an MI may cause hypotension yielding an early unfavorable outcome. If results in the first 12 hours were not counted, the initial adversity could have gone unrecognized.

Covariate Analysis

One can adjust the study groups to give equal representation for factors that can affect outcome by stratifying the groups. This can enhance balance between groups and correct outcomes that result from group imbalances. One can stratify at randomization, to correct for imbalances that can potentially affect outcome. However, this is not always possible. Only at the completion of a study may one arm of the study show an unintended imbalance in factors that can affect outcome. The effect of these factors on outcome can be re-balanced using methods of covariate analysis. Not all imbalances can be initially identified and knowing that they may affect outcome is often not possible when the study is planned. It is important to differentiate between covariates that are pre-specified at study initiation and those suspected at the time of analysis. Those identified late in the course of the study or at the time of analysis may introduce biases. Still a covariate analysis can be informative and should be carried out to correct a perceived imbalance.

If at the conclusion of study, analysis shows that there is an imbalance in a factor that may influence outcome, with that factor more prevalent in one of the arms of the study, then a covariant analysis should be undertaken with that factor as a covariant. The type of analysis depends on the covariate. If the covariate is discrete, a stratified analysis is performed such that the groups are stratified by the covariate for comparison. A comparison of the groups is made within each stratum and the results aggregated for a mean determination for the response variable, rebalancing the stratum for each treatment group compared to each control group. With a continuous response variable an adjustment for covariates is called an analysis of covariance. If one is analyzing a response variable by survival analysis, survival data can be evaluated by a Cox proportional hazard regression model with covariates varying with time. The more the covariates the greater the number of comparisons needed to correct the imbalance but this may potentially contribute to a Type I error.

Selection of covariates is based on prior knowledge, or a suspicion of what factors may influence outcome. Adjustments should be made for gender and age so that the study groups show balance, permitting an appropriate comparison. Other covariates may arise from the data review or knowledge of the disease being evaluated. One can try to adjust the response variable for other factors, such as a characteristic that correlates with a response to therapy or perhaps a marker for adherence. Adjusting for adherence to the protocol, health status or responding to therapy requires adjustment in the treated and untreated groups and the cause of the increased adherences, death status, or therapeutic responders may really be different due to the intervention between the two groups, and this can result in an inappropriate adjustment. These types of adjustments are controversial and need to be considered on a study-by-study basis, evaluating the rationale for undertaking the adjustment.

If the initial randomization is stratified, covariate analysis needs to be performed for those covariants. If the initial randomization is not stratified and the study is a large one, one may choose not to perform covariate analysis. Large studies often create balance in critical factors that may affect outcome. However, this is not always true and thus thought should be given to a covariate analysis, especially in disease states where covariates that affect outcome have been identified. As an example, diabetes increases the adverse outcomes in heart disease and a balance of patients with diabetes in the control and intervention group is appropriate. One may want to determine if there is a correlation between a covariate and outcome if the response to treatment varies with the covariate. This is called a treatment covariate interaction. The magnitude of the treatment effect can vary with outcome, or the treatment effect may be observed only at a specific level of treatment.

Survival Data Analysis

The primary outcome variable in many studies will compare the event rates in the treatment group to the event rate in the control group. This can be accomplished by comparing the event rates over a finite period of time as categorical variables, both in the treatment and control groups. But the rate of occurrence of the events may be different. In a cancer study the first-year mortality may be significantly less in the treatment group, while at five years the mortality may be the same. Prolonging the time to death can be considered a major treatment benefit and needs to be evaluated in an analysis of the study. The variable can be survival, or it can be the time to a significant event (myocardial infarction, defibrillation shock, hospitalization, etc.). One can construct a survival curve using a lifetable analysis. One can estimate the hazard rates as the number of events divided by the time at risk for an event. One can determine the hazard rates by parametric methods, but the hazard ratio may not be constant during the study, but a function of time thus employing an exponential model may not appropriately describe what is occurring. A non-parametric representation of survival is often employed. The commonest approach is the Kaplan-Meier method. One measures the time of entry into the study to the event for each patient. If the patient does not have an event, the patient is censored at the termination of follow up at study end. With a Kaplan-Meier lifetable the events, death and lost to follow up are tabulated with each event being tabulated at the time of occurrence. This can be grouped by having each event noted on the Y axis and the time to event on the X axis. Each event thus creates a stepwise decrement revealing the rate of events (a step function representation). From this curve a hazard rate can be determined. One can also estimate the median survival time if the population has been followed long enough such that half of the study participants have had an event. The survival curves of the treatment and the control groups can be compared for statistical significance by employing a Mantel-Haenszel statistic (log rank statistic). Additionally, as with other types of analysis, one can stratify using a covariate adjusted analysis. The analysis analyzes the two variables comparing them within each strata to determine if the results are consistent across strata. The Cox proportional regression model allows for analysis of survival data collected for discreet or continuous variables.

There are a number of programs available for survival analysis and Kaplan-Meier analysis with a plotting function and statistical significance evaluation.

Some examples are:

https://www.xistat.com/en/solutions/features/Kaplan-Meier-analysis

https://kmplot.com

https://www.jmp.com/free-trial

Some survival analysis calculation are:

https://astatsa.com/LogRankTest

https://www.easymedstat.com/kaplan-meier-survival-analysis-online-calculator

https://www.statkindom.com/kaplan-meier-html

Sensitivity Analysis

When analyzing a study, the question can arise as to what would be the outcome if the event numbers changed among groups. This can be especially important when the number of events are small, the significance is marginal or there has been problems with an excessive number of patients lost to follow up, are dropouts from the study, or there is considerable missing data. One can ask what if part or all of the missing endpoints were in the intervention group. Would that change outcome of the study? Could the study outcome have been influenced by the lack of data that may have been censored because the patient dropped out, or the patient was lost to follow up? This asks the question, is data excluded that argues against a positive outcome, or is data missing that if included could have resulted in a significant result? Showing that study results when counting missing events in an unfavorable way still results in a significant outcome adds credibility to the results. When reviewing data from pharmaceutical and device company applications to FDA, statisticians often perform a sensitivity analysis to evaluate the strength of a study's findings when an incomplete data set raises concerns with the study's conclusions.

A sensitivity analysis consists of inserting key outcome data that are missing in the data set either favoring a favorable outcome or detracting from significance of a given outcome. This can be done in a series of tests, incrementally introducing data that favors an outcome or data that is unfavorable to a given outcome. If a study found significance between the intervention arm and the control arm with 40 deaths in the intervention arm and 120 in the control arm with 20 missing patient outcomes in the intervention arm, one can perform a sensitivity analysis by assuming 5, 10, 15, or all 20 of the missing outcomes were deaths in the intervention arm. If all 20 missing outcomes are considered deaths and added to the intervention arm as deaths (60 deaths intervention and 120 deaths control) and one still finds significance, this analysis strongly supports the study conclusion. If the “tipping point” from significance to non-significance requires a small allocation of the missing outcomes for the intervention to no longer have a significant outcome, then the study conclusions are based on weak evidence and the findings suspect.

Heterogeneity of Treatment Effect

The variability of risks and/or benefits of an intervention reported in different patients is referred to as heterogeneity of treatment effect. In some patients the treatment may be quite effective, while in others it may be marginal or even ineffective. In the selection of a treatment, it is essential to know that the mean effect is beneficial. But the mean effect has a range and in some patients the treatment is not effective. A clinician wants to identify the treatment that will likely be effective in a given patient (his patient). The mean effect is less of interest. The clinician teats the individual patient however the mean effect is what is reported by most studies.

The determination of heterogeneity of treatment effect is often limited to the evaluation of pre-specified subgroups. The subgroups as we have discussed, are often small and thus any conclusions drawn are underpowered and thus inadequate to develop a sufficiently effective description to identify the extent of the beneficial treatment effect for individual patients. Additionally, the basis of identifying what constitutes most subgroups is one dimensional. Thus, it is unlikely that a subgroup will identify a factor that determines success or failure. The factor that might identify what constitutes the effectiveness of treatment such as a genetic subtype of disease are often not identified by subgroup analysis. Some have suggested (Kent et al Trial 2010:11:85) that the identification of the heterogeneity of treatment effect should be based on subgroups defined by multivariable risk and be quantified.

An alternative to the subgroup analysis approach is to employ a model that estimates the connection between multiple baseline characteristics that may explain outcome. The model assigns a multivariable risk score to each patient. One can use an existing risk prediction score derived from a study or a series of studies. Patients are divided into groupings of risks that correlate with a given treatment outcome. One can thus determine the extent to which a treatment success relates to the underlying characteristic components of the prediction score. A limitation of this approach is that the disease being evaluated may have multiple etiologies and thus the treatment may show a different response depending on the causation of the disease.

Another approach is to identify baseline factors that affect the effectiveness of the treatment. An interaction term can be estimated that relates treatment outcome and baseline factors. This effect model establishes how the average effect is modified by baseline factors. This approach works when the determinate of the success of the treatment effect has been measured in clinical trials. If the determinates are not measured, then the effectiveness model will not work.

In a paper by Kent and colleagues (Kent et al JAMA 2021:326(22), 2277-2286) the investigators identified two scales that identified patients at risk for a stroke when they have a Patent Foramen Ovalle (PFO). The risk of paradoxical embolism score (ROPE) and the PFO – Associated Stroke Causal Likelihood Classification System (PASCAL) assigned patients a risk score for a stroke. The investigators then used these scores based on a number in the trial who would benefit from a PFO closure. The score identified that there indeed is a heterogeneity of treatment effect. Patients with a high risk of stroke who had a PFO benefited from a surgical procedure to close the PFO, while those at low risk for a stroke had no benefit from a PFO surgical closure. Since there is a risk associated with the closure, there is considerable benefit in knowing who will show a reduction in stroke if the PFO is closed. A physician treating a patient with a PFO is assisted in determining stroke risk and thus the advisability of a surgical procedure to close the PFO. This is far more clinically useful than knowing that the mean effect of closing a PFO reduces stroke.

The use of measuring the heterogeneity of treatment effect and applying it to individualizing treatment decisions serves a considerable need in medicine and will be employed more frequently in future study reports to make the study results more useful in clinical practice.

Summary

There are many approaches to data analysis and establishing statistical significance. One can diligently undertake multiple analysis till one finds a way of confirming your hypothesis. However, it is far more appropriate to pre-specify the methods of analysis, the criteria for significance and then apply them to the study results. Unfortunately, studies don't often provide neat results. There are patients who drop out or change participation from one study arm to another. Patients in the best of studies can be lost to follow up. Despite aggressive efforts to determine the results of the primary variable in a given patient this may not be possible. Techniques are available to account for these problems still permitting a reasonable attempt at analyzing the study and determining the probability that the findings are significant. What is most important is to be forthcoming and explain in the statistical section of a paper how the results were analyzed, what assumptions were made with the data and how problems such as patients crossing over, lost to follow up and other missing information is handled. This will give support to one's results, establish the validity of the analysis and ensure that you make an honest contribution to the literature and clinical medicine.

Chapter 16. Trial Result Interpretation and Publication

The preparation of the results of a study for publication is an exciting time, the culmination of a lot of work and the hope that you have made a contribution to the field you have been studying. One needs to undertake the interpretation of the trial and preparing a publication with considerable planning. How the results of the trial are presented influences the acceptance of the results and its perceived value by the medical community. The paper needs to avoid over promotion of the results, avoid excessive speculation and avoid promoting trends and marginally significant results. Focus on the results relating to the primary research question. All additional findings will be more likely to be considered valid if the primary research question is positive and the null hypothesis rejected with a highly significant P value.

When a trial is evaluated by reviewers and by colleagues reading the paper the first consideration is the primary research question. Is it clearly stated and a reasonable hypothesis that has been evaluated in the study? Are the trial methods appropriate using validated techniques with validated tests instruments? Is the trial randomized and carried out correctly? Balancing the arms of the study for factors that can influence outcome gives validity to the findings. Were important covariates adjusted in the randomization process by employing a covariate analysis of the data? Is the sample size appropriate? If multiple comparisons are made, was this taken into account in the statistical plan? Were the appropriate statistics employed in the trial's analysis? Were secondary questions pre-specified in the trial and were they appropriately analyzed and was the sample size adequate to consider the secondary questions? Was the study appropriately controlled and blinded, limiting the potential for bias that can affect the results? Was the follow up period appropriate? Was the data set complete? Were patients lost to follow up or dropped from of the study? How were these problems dealt with in the study's analysis? Were there confounding effects of background therapy and if so, how were they taken into consideration in interpreting the results? Were the conclusions of the study fair, or is there bias affecting the reported results? Is there the potential for a conflict of interest? Is the introduction to the manuscript informative as to why the study was undertaken? Does the methods section explain how the study was performed so the readers of the manuscript can understand the methodology, its advantages and disadvantages? Does the discussion section of the paper discuss the study's findings and integrate them with reports published in the medical literature, further supporting the study conclusions? If the findings are at odds with other studies, why are the results contrary to other reports? How do the studies differ and what is the significance of the differences? Do the investigators clearly state the study's limitations and how the study's limitations may affect the results. These are some of the questions reviewers may raise in the review process and questions raised by one's colleagues when they read the paper.

Negative Studies

Some studies will present negative results. It is well known that positive findings are given priority for publication and positive findings are favored by reviewers. However, we are seeing more and more negative studies reported in major journals. Negative studies must overcome a publication bias. The reporting of negative studies is important for patient care and the advancement of medical science, often as much as are positive studies. If a study has negative findings one needs to evaluate if the sample size was adequate. It is critical that the authors state the power of the study when it was completed. Many studies do not have the power that was initially established when the initial sample size was determined. Were the outcome measurements sensitive to show a treatment effect? Assay sensitivity is an important consideration. When evaluating a negative study, one should always consider that the measuring technique(s) was not able to detect a difference among the study groups. In a study employing pharmacologic treatment; inadequate dose, inappropriate dosing intervals and at times inadequate duration of the therapy may be the explanation for a negative outcome.

The technical skills of the investigator may contribute to a negative study. If investigators perform few procedures "a learning effect" may not be overcome and may be an explanation for poor results. In a study on renal denervation on blood pressure lowering, the investigators had little experience with the difficult techniques of renal denervation. The failure to actually denervate the renal nerves in my estimation caused the study to report negative results. In studies with patient adherence problems, excessive “drop in” and “dropouts”, or patients lost to follow up causes the outcome to be uninterpretable or showing results that may be incorrect because of the missing data. How problems of adherence, study “drop ins”, “dropouts” or lost to follow up are handled in the data analysis are critical to an understanding of why a study may result in negative results. If imputation methods are employed, could they be used to explore possible causes of a negative outcome? Additionally, was the variance too high due to poor techniques, selection of an heterogeneous population or are outliers confounding the results, or were there competing events that the study endpoint did not take into consideration? Could have covariate adjustments been helpful in identifying factors that may transform a negative study into one that is positive? Would an analysis taking into account responders and excluding non-responders assist in understanding if treatment is effective or ineffective?

In a negative trial one may want to evaluate sub-groups that show a positive outcome. Not to claim that the trial is positive, but to generate a possible hypothesis that can be tested in future studies. This can enhance the study’s publication potential while not misleading the reader.

There are many factors that can affect trial results and the investigator must be vigilant as to possible confounding of the study. One should try to identify reasons for a study’s failure or reason to be suspicious of positive results, especially those that may be surprising in light of previous data. One example in the recent literature deals with drugs that lower triglycerides and thus reduce risk for coronary artery disease (CAD) development and progression. For years there has been little proof that pharmacologic agents that lower triglycerides actually reduce CAD. This is especially true for fish and fish oil products. The data that fish oil extract reduces CAD is very limited to nonexistent. Recently a study (REDUCE-it) reported that the omega-3 fatty acid concentrate icosapent ethyl (EPA) significantly lowered CAD risk (25%) compared to a placebo therapy (mineral oil) on top of standard medical therapy. Another trial of docosahexaenoic acid, another omega-3 fatty acid was compared to a placebo (corn oil) and showed no benefit on CAD events. One explanation for these findings is the perceptive insight of Dr. Steve Nissen who pointed out the difference in the comparative therapy (placebo) in the two trials. The mineral oil "placebo group" had a higher event rate than the DHA treated group, corn oil treated group as well as the EPA treated group. These findings suggest that the improvement in outcome was caused by the mineral oil treated group having increased CAD related events. In other words, the placebo may have been active with a negative effect on outcome. One conjecture then is that EPA was not beneficial but did no harm while the placebo arm did harm and thus increased the separation between events with EPA and the control group. While the details of these experiments may not be of interest to many, the example of how one explains contradicting results of large clinical outcome studies may be informative and help one to explain findings that may at first not be easily understood.

Consort Guidelines

For those who like a structured guideline on how to present data and the findings from a randomized blinded controlled trial with a checklist for optimizing the rigor of reporting, utilizing the Consolidated Standards of Reporting Trials (CONSORT) paradigm first published in 1996 with subsequent publication with revisions in 2001 and 2010 may be most helpful. The CONSORT guidelines can be very useful, especially for those new to the publication process. The CONSORT guidelines can be used as a reliable guide to what a credible paper should contain.

CONSORT 2010 Checklist

Section	Items
Title	Note if randomized trial
Abstract	Structured summary: method, results, conclusions
Introduction	Background & objectives
Methods	Trial design, participants, interventions, outcome measure, sample size, randomization, blind, statistical methods
Results	Participant flow diagram, recruitment, baseline data, intention to treat analysis, denominator of each group, outcomes with precision indicated, additional analysis of secondary questions, harms reported

Discussion	Limitations, generalizability, interpretation of results
Other	Registration, protocol outline, funding, conflict of interest

Registration

In planning a study, one should include a note that the study is registered. The need to register a study has come about due to several studies sponsored by corporate interests not being reported for outcomes that reported negative findings. This was alleged to be deliberate and thus registration was proposed to avoid the suppression of negative reports. Whether this is appropriate or not to require a registration process for clinical trials is moot, since to publish in most major Journals registration is requisite. Additionally, all studies sponsored by the government (NIH, NCI, etc.), all pharmaceutical and device studies that are under FDA supervision and review need to be registered. There are a number of possible registration sites, the most frequently employed is ClinicalTrials.gov. There is an initial form to be electronically completed that must be filed before the study is started. Once the study is complete there is a report that is required that contains a summary of the results of the trial. The registration process with ClinicalTrials.gov does take some time. The information reported becomes public knowledge. Many investigators, entrepreneurs and companies frequently review listings to offer services, develop competing products, or to keep tabs on a competitor's plans. Since the introduction of ClinicalTrials.gov, there have been a number of reports that the disclosure of study findings is often not done in a timely fashion and can be limited in the information revealed. There is controversy as to the need to increase information revealed and tightening of the timeline for reporting. The concept that clinical trial information should be in the public domain to increase medical knowledge of what works and what interventions may cause harm is unassailable. The timing of the release of this information is what remains in contention. Needless to say, not registering can limit the ability to publish and should not be omitted by an investigator for that very reason. When intellectual property concerns are raised it is appropriate to discuss matters with the intellectual property officer at one's academic institution, company, or with an intellectual property attorney. Issues of priority, whether a concept or therapeutic has already been in the public domain and thus precludes intellectual property protection can be most complicated to unravel and needs consideration by those expert in this area.

Chapter 17

The IRB In Clinical Research

The Investigational Review Board (IRB) or a Committee on Clinical Investigation is fundamental to the research process. The IRB's primary charge is to provide protection for patients participating in a study. The IRB aims to ensure the patient is properly informed of the risks involved in the study, the study procedures and the responsibilities of the investigators and their qualifications. The IRB ensures patients to be treated fairly and to be properly compensated, but not unfairly induced into participating in a study. The IRB is not there to evaluate the merits of the science or to facilitate clinical research. IRB's do evaluate the research in that a poorly organized study, one with no hope of reaching a positive conclusion, or one with a flawed research hypothesis is a study that poses risk to a patient with no benefit to the patient or society. Some academic research centers have a scientific committee to review the research, as well as an IRB to assess patient risk and advocate for patient rights. The IRB and clinical researchers must work together to initiate a clinical study, but the interest of the investigator in addressing a clinical hypothesis is less of a concern to an IRB than protecting the patient and ensuring a reasonable level of risk that a study poses to the patient.

It was not till the late 19th century that investigators began to obtain patient consent to perform clinical studies. Still many investigators would involve patients in studies with the patients not understanding the procedures or risks involved and without obtaining the patients agreement to participate. Patients were exposed to diseases in studies without their consent. Medical experiments sponsored by the German and Japanese governments in the 1940's were performed that caused pain, suffering and were outright torture. Often these studies caused the sadistic inflection of pain and death in the false guise of medical science. The United States government also sponsored studies that did not inform patients of existing and available alternative medical treatments to participating in a no treatment arm of a study. The CIA administered LSD to government employees and American citizens without their knowledge. This very unfortunate history led to the National Research Act in 1974 requiring an IRB review of research that was government sponsored. The Congress created a committee to generate a report on clinical research, the Belmont Report issued in 1979. The Belmont report was not adopted into law, but many of its recommendations became part of the 1981 amendment to Title 21 of Federal law, requiring IRB review of research. Most states also have requirements for research that includes an IRB review of research that is to be performed on humans before it may be initiated. The IRB is responsible to The Office of Human Research Protection (OHRP), a division of the Department of Health and Human Services. This office supervises IRB's. The common rule has been adapted by the U.S. government as a statement of the legal requirements for performing clinical research.

IRB Membership

There are rules for what constitutes an IRB. There must be members of both sexes at each meeting. There must be one member with a scientific background, one member without a scientific background on the committee and both must be at each meeting. If the IRB is affiliated with an institution, there must be at least one non-institutional affiliated member at each meeting. The potential conflicts of interests of each member must be made known and members of the IRB may not participate in a protocol review where a conflict may occur. There must be a minimum of 5 voting members at each IRB meeting and the meeting must be held with each member present in person. These are simple requirements, but unfortunately all IRB's do not always comply with these minimum requirements.

IRB Documentation

The IRB must have written procedures for its operation. All meetings must have minutes kept and records of all submissions, their review and all IRB actions documented, with all records maintained. All submissions to the IRB must be in writing, including submissions for the initial review, annual reports as well as for an expedited review. Any amendments to the protocol, any adverse reports and all correspondence with the IRB needs to be in writing and preserved by the IRB.

IRB Responsibilities

The primary responsibility of the IRB is to strive to ensure the safety of study participants. The IRB must evaluate the risk versus benefit that a study participant faces when taking part in the study. The IRB must judge the risk involved and if they are justifiable in light of the background information provided. The IRB must ensure that the potential study participant understands the risk of the study as explained in the consent form and its potential benefits, so the patient can make an informed decision as to whether to participate or not in the study. The procedures that a patient will undergo, the treatments received with their potential risk must be presented in a consent form approved by the IRB in language that a lay person can readily understand. The IRB is also charged with the responsibility of evaluating the scientific merit of a study, as to it being reasonable that the study will yield findings that justify subject participation with the inherent risks the study entails. The IRB is also charged with ensuring that the investigators are appropriately credentialed for the type of investigation they are conducting and that they have the experience and capabilities to bring the project to a timely and successful completion. The IRB must ensure that patient privacy and confidentiality of study findings are maintained.

The IRB Submission

The IRB submission consists of the study protocol, a patient consent form, the investigational brochure, patient information sheet(s), proposed patient reimbursements, honorarium, and any proposed advertising aimed at patient recruitment. The study protocol and what it contains has been discussed previously as well as the contents of the investigational brochure. Patient information sheets are often provided to guide the patient through the study, to provide appropriate contact information and emergency phone numbers.

The patient consent form is the primary document through which patients receive information about the study, its purpose, the risk and benefits, payments, and study procedures. The study consent has a series of sections that is straightforward and provide information about the study. The basic components of a consent are:

Purpose of study

Procedures that the study subject will undergo

The duration of the study

Where the study will be performed

Who are the investigators

Risks to the patient

Benefits to the patient

Patient alternatives other than participating in study

Patient information on privacy and confidentiality

Provisions for treatment of injury due to study participation

Financial responsibility for compensating patients for injuries during the study

Who to contact for questions or in case of an adverse reaction or emergency

Statement that participation is voluntary

Monetary reimbursement for patient incurred costs

Honorarium for patient participation

Place for signature of participant and witness of patient signing consent

Name of person taking consent and answering questions

Date and signature of patient

Most aspects of the consent are self-explanatory. Alternatives to participation should mention who the patient can turn to for medical care if patient chooses not to participate. A statement should be included in the consent that refusing to participant will not deny the patient appropriate medical care. A confidentiality statement should include that the patient will not be identified in any report that is derived from the study. The study consent should include a statement that the patient can withdraw form the study at any time by giving notice to the investigators. That all information obtained up to that point will remain in the study database. In some studies provisions can be granted in advance that the investigator may continue to obtain outcome measures on the patient even if the patient withdraws from the study. This follow up can be done if the patient initially gave consent for outcome measure follow up. This may include information on death and hospitalization. It is advisable that this release for long term follow up despite patient withdrawal be obtained in studies where outcome is a study endpoint. A statement is often included on who is financially responsible for emergency and long-term treatment if the patient is injured in the course of the study. Additionally, a statement is included that to receive treatment and potential compensation a patient must report the injury immediately to the study personnel. Most IRB's require that the investigator or sponsor of the study provide emergency care for patients for injuries sustained due to participation in the study. Follow up care and financial coverage of the cost of long-term care may be excluded in the consent form with IRB permission for this disclaimer. The expenses that the patient incurs that are reimbursable should be clearly outlined and when and how the payment is made. Many studies provide a stipend (honorarium) to the patient for the time they dedicate to the study. The amount offered is subject to IRB review and should not be of an amount that is a financial inducement for patient participation in the study. The amount offered should be accompanied by a statement that the stipend is amortized over the length of the study. If a patient withdraws after participating in half the study, the patient must receive half the stipend. The consent needs to be signed and dated by the study participant, witnessed by an individual not taking consent and not associated with the study and a copy of the consent needs to be given to the study participant. The person who takes the consent, who answers questions that the participant may pose needs to be identified as well.

Unfortunately, with the amount of information needed to be conveyed to the participant and the legal disclaimers often required by institutions (boiler plate material) a consent form may be as long as 5 to 25 pages. Patients rarely read the consent document and if one tries to read the document to them they often say they agree and don't want the long document read to them. Patients unfortunately often come away from the process without the critical information they should obtain from the consenting process. It would be optimum if consents could be shortened and especially consents offered to patient in emergency situations that are far shorter. A patient with acute chest pain thinking they are having a myocardial infarction can't really read through a 5- 25 page or longer document with the necessary degree of attention to understand the study. Unfortunately, the consent process is what it is. The investigator should at least review the highlights of the consent with the patient discussing alternatives, the critical risks that the patient may be taking and alternatives to study participation.

Obtaining Consent

There are a number of different consenting processes that can be employed. The standard is the written consent that the patient reads, and then study personnel answers any questions that may arise. The consent is then signed, and a copy given to the patient. If the study is with a child, the consent needs to be read and signed by the minor's legal guardian. If the subject is an adult, but not competent to sign a consent, then the patient's legal guardian must read and sign the consent. Children who understand what is happening should be explained orally the key elements of the consent and the investigator should obtain the assent of the minor as well as the guardian's written consent.

In emergency situations there can be a waiver of consent. This is for a condition where urgent care is required and the patient unable to give consent. Life-threatening situations such as a cardiac arrest, major trauma, head injury, or acute neurologic or psychiatric conditions can make consent unobtainable. To request waiver of consent one needs to survey the community's attitude to research and show that there is not a significant opposition to the research. One needs to show that the community and its leaders have been informed of the study and are not opposed. If a pharmaceutical or device is involved, then the FDA must approve that the conditions have been met for a waiver of consent and that the condition is one where the patient can't give consent and where current therapies are unsatisfactory or that the study therapy has potential to significantly improve upon the outcome expected with standard therapy. With IRB and FDA approval the study may commence without obtaining a written consent from the patient. However, each patient who is considered for the study must be evaluated by a physician independent of the study who agrees that the patient is appropriate to participate in the study. The independent physician must place a note in the patients record to that effect.

There is a provision for one time use of a waiver of consent. This is for an urgent situation where a patient may benefit from an experimental device or drug and there is no time for IRB review and approval. The intervention must be considered a potentially lifesaving one. The IRB chair may authorize a one-time emergency use. The physician should report the outcome to the IRB to be reviewed at a later date. If the physician wants to make use of the intervention subsequently, then a protocol and consent form should be developed and submitted for IRB review. Both for a medical device and pharmaceuticals that are not approved, the FDA has emergency use procedures if time permits. The FDA should be contacted by the investigator or sponsor of the drug or device before use. This is a onetime process and there is no justification for not making provisions for subsequent use if the device or drug is to be employed again.

There is also the process of a "partial disclosure consent". There are situations where the investigator may not want to inform the study subject all the information in the protocol. In this situation the investigator believes that the information if disclosed may affect the study outcome. These are usually psychology or psychiatry related studies. They must be of minimal risk and the IRB must be in agreement that full disclosure may alter study results.

There are studies such as chart reviews, retrospective data collection or employing established data bases where the investigators may request expedited review. An expedited review is for utilizing the data or collecting data from patients where there is no proposed consent process. Since there is no direct contact with patients and the data collection process does not alter patient care, a waiver of consent and expedited review can be requested. Some studies such as questionnaires or surveys may also fit into this category. An expedited review does not need a full committee review and can be granted by the IRB chair or designee. The IRB is generally informed of the expedited review granted at their next meeting.

The IRB Process

The initial contact with the IRB is the protocol and consent submission. The IRB reviews the protocol and consent and can approve, ask for modification, or turn down the proposal. After approval the investigator may commence the study. Often IRB's have questions regarding the study before approval and ask the primary investigator to appear before the committee for questioning. Investigators may appeal a denial of approval and ask the IRB to be present for an appeal. IRB's usually have a yearly reporting requirement, although some have semi-annual reporting requirements. In especially high-risk studies, the IRB may require reporting of study outcome after each patient entry, or after every few patients with the requirement that to proceed one needs IRB review and approval for the next patient (or group of patients) to be studied. The IRB and FDA may also audit a study. At the completion of the study the investigator must file a final report with the IRB. Each IRB will have guidance's on the information that needs to be reported. With multi-centered studies until the last few years each site needed to obtain approval from an IRB. Each institution would require its IRB to review the protocol. This duplication of work caused confusion and long delays. One IRB may request a protocol change, and this involved requiring approval from all the other site IRB's. Permitting a central IRB in multi-center trials in 2012 created a major paradigm shift, greatly facilitating clinical investigation. Multiple sites can employ a central IRB. Each site must obtain institutional permission to use the central IRB, but this is usually granted and greatly facilitates the IRB review process. Besides facilitating research this approach has removed the confusion of where to report adverse events. Omitting the need to obtain multiple approvals before a protocol initiation has greatly streamlined the multi-center research process.

Protocol Amendments

For many reasons a study protocol may need to be modified. These modifications take the form of amendments. Each amendment needs approval by the IRB. Unless the amendment causes major changes to the protocol or changes the risks and benefits the patient may encounter, the amendments are usually approved administratively by the IRB. Those amendments decided by the IRB chairperson that warrant full committee review will be reviewed and then voted on at the next IRB meeting. It is not usual for studies to have dozens of administrative amendments and occasional full committee review requiring amendments.

IRB Reporting

The investigator must report to the IRB all serious adverse

reactions. Expected adverse reactions, those described in the investigator brochure need to be reported at specified reporting intervals. However, some IRB's require any serious adverse event that may be related to the study to be reported to the IRB. The code of federal regulation states "that reporting study endpoints (e.g. mortality or major morbidity - hospitalization, disability, etc.) described in the protocol and the Investigational Brochure that are expected can be reported to the FDA in the annual report. "However, if a serious and unexpected adverse event occurs for which there is evidence suggesting a causal relationship between the drug (or device) and the event, the event mut be reported". Some IRB's may go further and request all deaths and hospitalizations be reported to the IRB, regardless of relation to the study and despite the study being designed essentiality to accumulate these endpoints that result from the disease process. IRB's often confuse adverse reports with study endpoints. The reporting plans of the study should be conveyed to the IRB in advance by a clear statement in the protocol or the Data Monitoring and Privacy Plan, a plan that is now often required by IRB's in addition to the traditional protocol, consent and Investigative Brochure.

Chapter 18
The U.S. Drug Development Process

The U.S. regulatory authority over drug development and approval is through the Food and Drug Administration (FDA) which is part of the U.S. Department of Health and Human Services. From the very start of government regulation of pharmaceuticals the urgency of regulation has been forced upon Congress by emergencies and scandals that have precipitated action. From food additives in the 1830's, vaccine contamination in the early 1900's to the elixir sulfonamide and radiothon precipitating the 1938 Food Drug and Cosmetic Act, Congress has legislated by reaction to crises. The authority to regulate drug development on the basis of drug efficacy was fully granted to FDA with the 1962 Drug Amendments following the Kefauver Hearing and the reports of phocomelia due to Thalidomide. Today the regulatory process of drug development is well codified.

The FDA is headed by a commissioner appointed by the President and confirmed by the Senate. This Commissioner of FDA has multiple deputies. The entity having jurisdiction over drugs is CDER (Center for Drug Evaluation and Research) and for medical device development it is CDRH (Center for Device and Radiologic Health). There is a Center for Biologic Evaluation and Research (CBER), but most of the approvals of biologic agents are now through CDER with vaccines and arcinials approval still through

CBER.

The Drug Development Process consists of drug discovery, formulation development and pre-clinical work performed by a sponsor. This work is then submitted together as an application to the FDA for an IND (Investigational New Drug). The IND is essentially a waiver to transport and study an investigational drug in interstate commerce in the U.S. Following the granting of an IND, the sponsor then can embark on clinical studies which can be divided into four stages. Stages I through III are required to be completed to submit an application for approval of a new chemical entity for distribution and sale in the U.S. The application is called an NDA (New Drug Application). CDER has multiple divisions that deal with specific areas. A drug for cardiac disease for example, would obtain the IND and subsequent NDA through the Cardio-Renal Division of FDA. The appropriate division reviews the NDA application and makes a recommendation to the Division Head. FDA may decide to convene a panel of advisors which they often do for new chemical entities being reviewed for an NDA. These advisors comprise a standing committee called an FDA Advisory Committee, though FDA may call upon ad hoc advisors. The committee hears an FDA presentation and one from the sponsor. The committee asks questions both to the FDA and sponsor and then discusses issues raised and then makes a recommendation. FDA may or may not follow the recommendations of an advisory committee. The relevant FDA division director then makes a recommendation, which then goes to the CDER director or his designee, who will recommend to the commissioner whether to approve, deny, or request additional data for drug approval. Once a drug is approved there may be post-approval studies mandated for additional information or studies aimed at improving marketing prospects of the drug, both types of studies are characterized as Phase IV studies. The sponsor must provide periodic reports to FDA and maintain an adverse event surveillance system. Some drugs that are approved have risks posed by the drug that are of such a high risk that FDA can mandate a limited, controlled distribution of the drug. These limitations for distribution often involve risk mitigation strategies (REMs). If an approved drug has efficacy in a similar or an unrelated area that differs from the approved indications the sponsors must develop the drug for these new indications and needs to obtain a new IND, submit a new or supplemental NDA and proceed through the approval process for the new indication. An example would be a drug approved for the treatment of hypertension. The drug's actions suggest it would also be a useful for the treatment for heart failure. To obtain a heart failure claim, the sponsor would need to file a new IND, undertake studies in heart failure, and then proceed to file a second NDA.

Pre-Clinical Studies

The drug development process often starts with drug discovery of new chemical entities (NCE). The drug development process can take 10-12 years costing 800 million to 2 billion dollars. Some estimate that out of 4,000 drug candidates 3,999 fail to reach approval. If 100 compounds progress through the discovery and pre-clinical screen usually only one goes on to clinical trials. Of ten compounds that make it to clinical trials perhaps one succeeds to be marketed. Out of 100 compounds that are marketed one might be a blockbuster that will support a large pharmaceutical company that has so many failures in the development process. Drug development is very capital intensive, and the very high cost of pharmaceuticals is in part the result of the cost of maintaining a process where so few products are profitable, guaranteeing a return on investment commensurate with other investment opportunities.

The initial efforts for drug discovery can be undertaken with a directed process that takes into account disease pathophysiology and the biochemistry behind the disease. An alternative development of NCEs may be based on combinational chemistry, creating thousands of compounds that must be run through drug screens to determine potential candidates. What one screens for is what one will find. For example, if one screens for potential anti-arrhythmic agents to suppress extra ventricular beats (VPC's), one may not find a drug that suppresses ventricular tachycardia or stabilizes the heart from developing ventricular fibrillation. The screen will determine the type of drug one identifies and might choose to develop. Once a compound is identified, then more involved physiologic experiments need be considered to evaluate the drug's physiologic effects. In vivo dose assessments, toxic dose levels and dosing intervals needs to be established. As a candidate compound appears more promising, long-term toxicology, teratogenicity, and immunogenicity studies, along with drug metabolism studies will be initiated (ADME studies: absorption, distribution, metabolism and elimination). Reproductive toxicology and carcinogenicity studies will also be needed. While some argue that all these evaluations can be done in vitro without animal experimentation this is **not** true and to bypass animal studies would severely limit drug discovery and markedly increase risk to humans exposed to experimental therapies. When a new candidate drug has demonstrated efficacy against the target disease in pre-clinical studies and an initial acceptable safety signal is established one would then proceed to a clinical evaluation.

IND Process

To proceed to clinical trials a sponsor must obtain an IND (Investigational New Drug) designation. This permits the sponsor to initiate clinical studies. The FDA can regulate drugs engaged in interstate commerce and an IND waives the need for approval to ship study drugs among the 50 states and thus the capability to evaluate an unapproved drug. One might believe that if all the studies were done in one state, an IND would not be required. However, FDA has a very broad definition of interstate commerce, so if any component of the drug, any part of the container any manufacturing, any part of the study is outside a single state, an IND is needed. For all intent and purpose, all drug development requires an IND.

The IND can be obtained by a commercial sponsor, but an IND can also be obtained by an academic investigator who may be utilizing an experimental drug in a research project. There may be less requirements for an investigator IND than a commercial IND.

Investigators should not perceive the IND process as a daunting, impossible process. There are also treatment and compassionate use IND's for drug therapies not currently approved. FDA may exempt a drug from IND requirements if all of the following conditions are met: (1) The study is not for a medical indication or new product label, (2) The study using the agent is not intended for FDA submission, (3) There are no dose changes from an approved version of the drug and (4) IRB approval is obtained for the study in which the drug will be employed.

The IND contains the following sections: chemistry manufacturing and control information (CMC), drug characterization and identification, quality control, purity, and strength of the drug. The sponsor or investigator needs to supply a 1571 form – updated version 2012 that describes the information being provided and intended use of the drug, a 1572 statement of qualifications of the investigator and to provide sponsor and FDA with required information to evaluate a specific agent. In addition, a proposed trial needs to be listed in ClinicalTrials.gov with evidence of registration. The contents of an IND is listed in Table I.

Table I: IND Contents

FDA Form #1571

FDA Form #1572

Drug Substance Description

Manufacturing Methods

Methods of Preparation

Analytical Methods

Validation Procedure

Stability Data

Packaging Description

Sterility (if appropriate, i.e. intravenous formulations)

Microbiology

Pyrogenicity

Label for packaging

Pharmacology – pre-clinical

Toxicology

Environmental Impact Statement

Initial (Index) Protocol

Investigator Brochure

Once an IND is filed, the FDA has 30-days to review. If one does not hear form FDA in 30-days, the sponsor or investigator may proceed. The sponsor or investigator should provide an initial protocol for the planned first study (Index Protocol). The Investigator Brochure contents is described in Table II. Each subsequent clinical study needs to be submitted under the IND for FDA review and 30-days must elapse before one can proceed with the study unless FDA requires more information or additional review time. FDA may ask for an IND meeting to discuss the proposal or FDA may make suggestions for changes to meet FDA standards for an IND or to modify the proposed clinical study. There are IND's that are rejected by FDA, or the FDA may request further pre-clinical studies (efficacy, safety, or both) before the IND is re-considered.

Table II Investigator Brochure

Sponsor

Product Name

Chemical Name

Summary

Background

Physical, chemical, pharmacologic properties

Formulation Information

Non-Clinical Studies:

- In vitro pre-clinical
- In vivo pre-clinical
- Pharmacokinetic
- Metabolic
- Safety
- Efficacy
- Toxicology
- Clinical Observation Outside U.S. Experience

Publications

Protocols underway or planned

Clinical Trials I-IV

A drug development plan aims to receive approval of an NDA. To gain approval the NDA must contain 2 pivotal clinical trials that are randomized, most often blinded, that have a control arm. Prior to these pivotal trials there are often dose ranging studies and then initial efficacy studies. All these trials constitute the clinical part of the development program. The development program can be divided into four phases. Phase I trials are first in man studies. They measure physiologic variables (BP, HR), determine initial safety and may be used to obtain the first kinetic data in man. Often generic drug studies comparing pharmacokinetics of a proprietary drug and its imitator are also called Phase I studies. When very potentially toxic drugs are first evaluated, such as anti-neoplastic agents, patients will be utilized as opposed to routine pharmacokinetic studies and generic drug bioequivalence studies where normal volunteers are employed.

Phase II studies are small studies evaluating the short-term effects of a drug, usually on physiologic endpoints. They are employed to give an initial signal of drug efficacy, show toxicity that can be observed early on and also to help determine optimum dosing. Those studies are usually blinded, crossover and placebo controlled.

Phase III studies are the pivotal trials in the development program. They are usually blinded, randomized, often stratified and usually employ a parallel design. These trials are used to establish efficacy with natural history endpoints and to determine safety of prolonged drug administration. The studies usually last a year or two for the length of each patient's follow up. Often these studies are expanded after completion to "open label" studies where patients may receive prolonged drug administration for compassionate reasons as well as to obtain long-term safety information. These studies may extend beyond the NDA submission and transition into Phase IV trials.

Phase IV studies by definition are studies after the NDA is submitted. They can be comparative efficacy studies, with the study drug compared to similar established treatments. They may be trials to establish equivalence, or non-inferiority to alternative therapies, or to explore new dosing regimens or possible drug interactions. These studies compare the drug under study to a positive control of an established therapy(s). Phase IV studies may also explore the effect of the drug in different populations, more severe (or less severe disease), or may evaluate the drug in special populations.

Some development programs follow a very traditional outline with Phase I studies of kinetics in normal volunteers, Phase II crossover efficacy trials of study drug vs. placebo possibly with a forced titration component. Phase III trials are usually of a parallel design evaluating safety and efficacy and Phase IV are often drug comparative studies. Other programs may have Phase I trials in patients, Phase II efficacy and early safety studies using biomarkers (either crossover or parallel design studies) with subsequent Phase III positive control natural history endpoint, parallel design studies. Phase IV trials may be undertaken in less ill patients, comparing efficacy in select populations and to determine superiority to standard of care therapy. Phase I studies usually consist of a few dozen patients with little attempt to determine sample size with the use of power calculations. These are short trials lasting a day to a week. Phase II studies last several months to a year and contain up to several hundred patients using physiologic or biomarker endpoints. Phase III studies may consist of hundreds to thousands of patients, followed for a couple of years and employ endpoints such as survival and hospitalization, categorical, natural history endpoints.

The NDA Application

The NDA application builds upon the IND submission. Additional pre-clinical studies have been completed, new toxicology studies have been undertaken and often with results extending for a year or two. Manufacturing methods have been refined along with analytical procedures. Stability has now been determined for 1-2 years and package labelling for marketed drug completed. This new information with summaries of the Phase I – III clinical studies will now constitute the NDA.

NDA Application

FDA 356h Form

Index

Summary

Proposed package insert – referenced to supporting data in NDA (annotated)

Manufacturing, controls, methods validation

Pre-Clinical pharmacology, toxicology, metabolism, kinetics

Microbiology

Clinical Data

Statistical Report

Case Form and Tabulation of Pivotal Studies

Safety Summary

Risk Benefit Ratio Discussion

Patent Certification

Debarment Statement

The clinical studies section starts with Phase I bioavailability and pharmacokinetic studies. Then the Phase II controlled clinical trials followed by the Phase III pivotal studies. One can also provide data obtained from uncontrolled studies, studies performed outside the U.S. and any other safety studies, or reports obtained on the drug product. Studies in special populations are also reported. A safety summary is included, listing adverse events (best to have study results from studies that compare drug to placebo). Relevant clinical lab data (hepatic, renal, hematologic) needs to be submitted. Any information on overdosage, problems in special populations and any reports on abuse potential. There should also be a discussion of the risk benefit ratio of the drug and why the drug should be acceptable given the disease state being treated. The entire presentation needs to be in the context of the requested indication for approval. The clinical findings, the safety reports and the risk benefit ratio need to be discussed in terms of the specific indication that the drug is being considered for approval. A cancer drug with severe toxicity is often approved if it improves survival in a clinically meaningful way despite very significant organ toxicities. An antihistamine that prolongs the QT and may give rise to life-threatening cardiac arrhythmias will not be approved even if it is the best antihistamine ever synthetized with no other reported toxicities in man. A drug with no reports of adversity in controlled studies may not receive approval if in pre-clinical studies it is a potent and extensive inhibitor of the P450 (CYP) hepatic enzyme system given FDA's experience with mibefradil.

Regulatory Considerations

A product application needs to be classified. It can be a new chemical entity, a new salt of the entity, a new formulation of an already approved drug, a new combination drug, an already marketed drug for a new indication, or a reformulated drug of an already approved drug. A drug can undergo a standard review or a priority review and this must be requested at the time of NDA submission or prior to the submission. The IND and NDA material may be complete, or if applicable the sponsor can submit a request under section 505(b)2 of the Federal Code, requesting that missing components of the NDA be reviewed from FDA internal files of another drug product submitted previously to FDA that is very similar or the same as the drug under consideration. For instance, the toxicology from an oral anti-arrhythmic may be cross referenced and sited in a submission of an IV formulation of that drug under the 505(b)2 request. Thus, the IV drug submission may not contain independent toxicology studies.

When an NDA is filed, FDA may accept the filing, request additional information, reject the NDA filing on the basis of being incomplete – a refuse to file notice, or let the application proceed. The FDA reviewers may pose questions regarding the submission or ask for additional information or specific revisions of specific sections. The division reviews the application and can request an FDA Advisory Committee Meeting. During this process the sponsor may submit updates (amendments) to the NDA. During the review the sponsor submits safety reports at 4 months and quarterly thereafter. FDA may accept the NDA with an approval letter, an approval letter listing deficiencies that needs to be addressed before final approval or issue a non-approval letter. A non-approvable letter may be appealed. Often the FDA may also specify additional information needed before consideration for approval or post-approval studies that will be required. Post approval studies don't facilitate approval but are needed for the safe and effective use of the drug in the future. The findings of post-approval studies may be added to the product insert at a later date with FDA approval. The FDA may penalize a sponsor for not performing post approval studies and can even withdraw drug approval, though this penalty has not been applied.

There is one FDA drug development statute that is useful for clinical investigators to know. That is the Orphan Drug statute. This was developed to facilitate development and approval of drugs for conditions that affect small numbers of patients. Drugs benefiting conditions affecting small numbers of patients notoriously in the past made drug development less attractive to "big pharma". Academic investigators can operate in this space since the requirement for FDA "user fees" are waived, the FDA provides assistance at all levels of the process and FDA may require a single clinical study for approval with a very limited number of patients. An Orphan Drug is defined as a drug for a disease which affects 200,000 patients or less a year in the U.S. The benefits of an orphan drug designation are 7 years exclusivity, regardless of patent status, the possibility of an FDA grant to assist in the clinical study (very few awarded), and FDA assistance in IND and NDA preparation. Often only one pivotal trial is required for drug approval. Orphan Drug developers receive a 50% tax credit on development expenses. The Orphan Drug application is a separate process and must be submitted before the NDA is submitted. The Orphan Drug Designation if granted is listed in the public domain. There are certain statutory requirements that come with the designation; the most significant is a 1-year notice before a sponsor can discontinue the drug. Once the NDA is approved the Orphan Designation becomes exclusive to the holder. Another sponsor can obtain an Orphan Designation for a similar or the same drug if the sponsor shows safety or efficacy superiority to the prior approved agent.

FDA Priority Review Voucher Program

Priority review vouchers are an incentive program authorized by Congress to facilitate the development of treatments for underfunded, neglected, or rare diseases. A sponsor bringing to market a new drug treatment in designated areas will receive a voucher from FDA ensuring expedited review of another drug at a later date. The expedited review is for a second drug that may not be in an area of an underfunded, neglected, or treating, a rare disease. The priority review shortens the FDA's decision deadline to six months. The voucher program is part of the 2007 Food and Drug Administration Amendment Act (FDAAA). Initially the program dealt with tropical diseases, the program later expanded to include rare pediatric disease. In 2022 the company BioMarin, sold its Priority Review Voucher for $110 million. The legislation authorizing the voucher program periodically needs reauthorization by FDA and the program may not be continued though it has been very successful as an incentive for rare disease drug development.

Chapter 19

The US Medical Device Development

The medical device approval process is a convoluted one because the regulation of medical devices came later than drugs and the approval and oversight role of FDA was developed through a series of compromises in the Congressional legislative process. The regulation of medical devices and their approval process starts with the 1976 Medical Device Amendments. Devices on the market before 1976 are pre-amendment devices and these devices were to remain on the market. Devices not on the market before 1976 are termed post amendment devices and are subject to FDA review according to their classification.

Medical devices are instruments, apparatus, implements, machines, implants, reagents that are employed in the medical field. Class I devices are simple devices such as gauze pads or tongue depressors. They require facility regulation, product testing, and a pre-market notification to FDA. Class I devices must follow good manufacturing practice (GMP) in their production and are subject to quality system regulation (QSR). Class II devices are more complex devices and can range from ECG machines, surgical drapes, or electrocautery machines as examples. They need to establish safety and efficacy beyond what is needed for Class I devices. The Class II devices must meet performance standards that go beyond general controls. There is a requirement for a Class II device to report their use in patients as would be the case with patient registries. They can require pre-market review, but often don't. Class III devices are life-sustaining devices, or devices that if malfunction may be life-threatening. An example would be a pacemaker, heart-lung machine, or a cardiac valve implant. Class III devices need pre-market approval. There are also custom devices made for individual use such as orthopedic shoes that are not classified, are not registered and do not need FDA approval.

There are two major pathways for the approval of medical devices, excepting Class I devices which are exempt. There is the 510 K pre-market notification pathway, or the PMA (pre-market approval) pathway. The 510 K pathway is suitable for Class II and some Class III devices. It requires a 90-day notification to FDA prior to marketing. If FDA objects, the product is not marketed and subject to FDA review and the possible request by FDA for further evaluation and even clinical testing. 510 K devices must be "substantially equivalent" to a pre-market device or may contain functional aspects of multiple pre-market devices. A pacemaker available before 1976 is a very different device than one developed in 2022. But there is a pre-market device that a sponsor can utilize as a predicate to which they can compare their device. The sponsor can file a 510 K application giving a 90-day notice for FDA to decide if the device can go on the market without further studies. Class III devices are required to have a PMA filed before marketing. Additionally, FDA can and has at times called for a PMA study for a Class II or III device that has a predicate prior to 1976, but in the opinion of FDA warrants a PMA. This can be appealed by a sponsor. If the approval is denied these devices then can't file for marketing under the 510 K regulations. It is interesting to note that three-quarters of all medical devices are marketed through the 510 K process. The 510 K process is a far simpler pathway for a medical device to enter the marketplace than the PMA pathway.

PMA development is primarily for Class III devices. The PMA pathway requires pre-clinical testing and clinical studies (usually one) to establish safety and efficacy of the device in a clinical setting. Manufacturing methods, facility regulation, manufacturing controls and pre-clinical testing are all prerequisites before a clinical trial can commence. The FDA must approve an investigational authorization to initiate clinical trials called an Investigational Device Exemption (IDE). For a device to receive approval the sponsor must draft an IFU (instructions for use) which serves for medical devices as the package insert does for pharmaceutical products. The claims in the IFU must be substantiated by the clinical study that has been undertaken with the device. An alternative to the PMA pathway is the PDP (product development protocol) which involves FDA early in the development plan with ongoing planning and testing of the device. FDA participants in the planning and evaluation of study results with the device. The PDP program is seldom used by industry. A sponsor can request a down classification of a device from a Class III to a Class II, exempting the device from the need for a PMA. The congressional mandate to FDA is that the device review process must use the least burdensome pathway to facilitate the approval process.

At times FDA has called for a hybrid 510 K pathway for approval with a 510 K application, requesting the application to include clinical trial data. Data substantiating the clinical equivalence to the marketed predicate device or clinical safety data for approval can be required. This is not a request for a clinical trial per se but for clinical experience with the device; information as to device's safety and at times effectiveness.

As the Orphan Drug Law facilitates development of drugs for rare infrequent medical conditions there is the HDE (humanitarian device exemption) to facilitate device development for rare conditions. For an HDE, the condition for use must be less than 4,000 patients in number per year. When an HDE application is filed, the FDA has 75 days to respond to the sponsor as to whether the device qualifies for an HDE.

Device Studies

A device sponsor will test a Class III device in vitro developing in vitro safety data and information on reliability of the device (performance characteristics). Many groupings of devices have established testing procedures and existing performance standards. A developer will submit this information to FDA with a request for an IDE (investigational device exemption) to evaluate the device in man. The IDE is analogous to the IND for drugs. The sponsor will then organize a clinical study to determine efficacy and provide safety information on the device. The trials are usually parallel design with a comparative arm of standard care. Blinding a device therapy study is far harder than for a drug. At best many of the studies blind the evaluators who may evaluate questionnaires or compiled clinical outcome data. The studies need to be randomized, need to be balanced and need to include patients that will be treated once the device is marketed, providing generalizable results. Device studies usually have a year's follow up, through devices that have a significant impact on the patient's survival may be studied for longer periods and in far greater numbers (often post approval). While device studies may only have a few hundred patients, studies with devices such as cardiac stents or transvenous delivered heart valves have consisted of thousands of patients with a couple of year's follow up. It is common for device studies to employ composite endpoints to reduce the sample size while maintaining power. Studies with devices are usually multi-centered involving many investigators. Having a diversity of operators gives information on the influence of operator experience on the success and safety of the device. With devices there may be a "learning curve" such that the operator becomes more experienced as the number of cases increases and thus effectiveness and safety increases. For this reason, some trials will have a "blanking period" or "run in" where the outcomes of the first few cases are not counted because the operator is "learning" how to use the device and the study aims to evaluate the safety and efficacy of the device and not the device operator interaction. Censoring a learning period result can be appropriate, but the information obtained from the first few cases will be informative as to how the device should be released and what training may be necessary for physician operators. A device approval might require proctor session by an expert to instruct new users on the device so that new operators who are approved use the device safely with the effectiveness as determined in the clinical study. Information obtained during the “learning period” may be very useful for the writing of the IFU and a user manual.

Device studies are difficult to blind, though without blinding bias can be introduced into the study. If at all possible, a sham procedure should be utilized to facilitate blinding. In a study on the use of renal nerve ablation to reduce arterial blood pressure, the introduction of a sham procedure led to the finding of no significant differences in BP lowering between ablated and non-ablated patients. This was very different from previous studies that did not employ a sham procedure. Some believed that the patient knowing whether they received the ablation or not effected the blood pressure results of the study. However, it is now generally accepted that the lack of appropriate ablation skill of the operators and thus lack of renal nerve denervation, led to the negative study outcome. Still if at all possible and if ethical, a sham procedure to blind a device study is recommended.

The Review Process

The Center for Device and Radiologic Health (CDRH) first reviews a PMA submission. The review team may request more information or make an evaluation and submit the determination to the division director. New, novel devices, devices that may pose considerable risk or devices posing difficult questions to the reviewers during consideration can be presented to an Advisory

Committee. The committee hears both the sponsor and FDA presentations, deliberates and makes a recommendation. FDA may or may not follow the recommendation to approve the device for marketing. FDA may ask for further studies or decline approval. Once approved the sponsor may be required to perform post-approval studies. These studies are not to substitute for studies needed to gain approval, but to provide additional information that may further inform uses of the device on its long-term effectiveness, its safety or its use in populations that may not have been studied initially. Additionally, the sponsor may initiate studies to further introduce the device to the medical field or compare the device to a competitor's device for marketing purposes.

Device Event Monitoring

Adverse device reporting is done through the Med Watch program. Based on sponsor reports and reports in Med Watch, FDA may order a device recall. There are three classes of device recalls, Class I recalls being the most significant recalls for potentially life-threatening problems. Recalls are reported to the Manufacturer's and User Device Experience (MAUDE) data base maintained by FDA. MAUDE information is being incorporated in a more comprehensive data base, National Evaluation System of Health Technology (NEST). This system is intended to improve real time availability of information on device safety.

The incidence of Class I recalls is significantly greater for cardiovascular and surgical devices that are approved through the 510K pathway than those approved through a PMA. This suggests that the PMA process identifies more problematic devices than does the 510K process before marketing of the device and thus the PMA process provides greater safety to the public for the approval of devices. This is true despite the fact that PMA devices are by definition have a greater potential for life-threatening outcome, further supporting the thesis that more extensive pre-clinical and clinical studies identify safety issues before approval.

Chapter 20

Innovation in Clinical Research

In clinical research one often formulates the clinical research question based on prior research. We may set out to determine if a procedure or device is effective in a given clinical condition and if it is superior or non-inferior to alternative approaches. There are important clinical research questions and a systematic approach to carry out this research will certainly advance evidenced based medicine. There are other dimensions to clinical research that are innovative. One can develop a new approach to a disease treatment, or a new way to solve a clinical problem that may be novel and that offers considerable benefit. Innovative research may offer new therapeutic approach that can be of considerable benefit to patients.

To be innovative one must be a keen observer. One needs to thoroughly understand a clinical problem. One must try to simplify the situation to give insight to alternative approaches. The alternatives should be formulated in the form of a hypothesis that can be tested. Often one first evaluates a novel approach with a "proof of concept" study and then subject the concept to a more definitive proof with more extensive pre-clinical studies and further clinical trials.

Keys to Innovation

There are some important considerations to facilitate

innovation. Be skeptical, don't easily accept the prevailing view or the dominant approach to a disease treatment. As a resident I recall being severely criticized for treating a patient with hypertension who was having an acute MI with a beta blocker. The prevailing view was that a beta blocker would cause hypotension and thus would worsen a patient's condition. However, Dr. Swedberg among other Scandinavian clinicians were treating patients having a myocardial infarction with beta blockers to good effect. Why would someone withdraw a beta blocker from a patient having an MI who is tachycardiac and hypertensive? Well, it's obvious, prevailing medical opinion was that the beta blocker would cause hypotension and thus "rob" the heat of circulation it needed when suffering from an acute MI. Contrary to prevailing opinion, clinical studies have subsequently demonstrated a mortality benefit of beta blocker therapy in the setting of an acute MI. Avoid "group think" and challenge orthodoxy. These are the watch words of the innovator.

Another key to innovation is to bring new expertise to a clinical problem. Use expertise and advances in science from other fields and apply them to the clinical problem at hand. Creating an RNA vaccine for COVID came from RNA technology that was being targeted to other clinical problems. Utilizing technologies from the basic sciences and applying these advances to clinical problems in very different areas may create innovative solutions. A clinical researcher with expertise in another area may pose an innovative hypothesis based on knowledge not available to others in the field. An example was the ability to determine the degree of stenosis of cardiac aortic valves with the hemodynamic data obtained at a cardiac catheterization. A cardiology fellow at the time, Dr. Richard Gorlin, turned to his father a fluid dynamic engineer to help in the discovery of the Gorlin formula for valve area. Knowledge of molecular biology, chemistry, engineering, computer science may offer new approaches to clinical medicine. One needs to be open to different approaches to problems in fields that are thought to be settled. There is often room for improvement in therapeutics with the goal of reducing toxicity of a treatment and improving efficacy.

The solutions to clinical problems may be complex, but one should strive to simplify. The more complex the project the more likely to fail. The more therapeutic modalities in use, the more likely toxicities will develop, and the treatments will fail. One needs to strive for a simplified approach and a research question that can be addressed as simply as possible if one hopes for a breakthrough. This is not advocating a simplistic, pollyanna approach, but addressing complex processes with simpler approaches that solve a problem. I have always admired the revolutionary approach of Dr. Barry Marshal to the understanding of peptic ulcer disease. Dr Marshal, a clinical gastroenterologist didn't accept that gastric ulcers resulted only from high acid levels. He questioned the accepted orthodoxy and came across autopsy pathologic studies showing bacteria in the stomach of ulcer patients. Believing an infectious etiology of gastric ulcer disease was a "far out" idea, but one that has been definitively proven and the basis of revolutionary therapy, markedly reducing morbidity and mortality.

I had the good fortune to spend an evening with Dr. John Black who made revolutionary discoveries with the B_1 and B_2 receptors and was able to develop drugs that had either more B_1 or B_2 agonist properties. He then went on to discover H_1 and H_2 receptors and pharmaceutical agents that blocked one or the other receptor. I asked Dr. Black how he was able to make such important insights not once, but twice in his career. He responded that it was "easy". With beta blockers he saw that different agents had slightly different degrees of effect on heart rate, blood pressure, or airway flow. This suggested to Dr. Black that different subsets of receptors were involved in different tissues revealing different degrees of agonist action. This was again seen with antihistamines having varied effects in different tissues and thus the presence of receptor subtypes was postulated. This led to the synthesis of several selective agents. These examples come from two gifted physicians who won the Nobel Prize for their insights. Most of us don't expect to make such profound breakthroughs or win a Nobel. But innovation can occur at all levels, making important contributions and improving patient care and patient outcomes. In the Masters in Clinical Research Course I taught and directed at Rush University for 21 years, I held a workshop on innovation with our residents, fellows and junior faculty. Let me present two of the workshop examples from my career that may be informative.

Innovation Workshop: The IV Sotalol Problem

Sotalol is a Type III anti-arrhythmic agent that is also a beta blocker. Type III anti-arrhythmic agents prolong cardiac repolarization which is reflected on the ECG as QT prolongation. Many Type III anti-arrhythmics can cause arrhythmias as well as effectively treating arrhythmias. Some agents such as amiodarone prolongs the QT but very rarely causes arrhythmias. However, sotalol has a 3 to 6% incidence of causing serious arrhythmias and this is much higher if the patient's heart function is weak due to myocardial disease (heart failure). Thus, when starting a patient on sotalol to prevent atrial fibrillation from re-occurring patients are admitted to a hospital under continuous ECG monitoring for 3 days till the full effects of sotalol are given time to affect the QT. Those who show excessive QT prolongation during this observation period have the sotalol therapy stopped. However, if a patient has a serious arrhythmia, it will take days for the sotalol levels in the blood to significantly diminish. I developed an IV sotalol formulation to make the loading phase shorter. With an IV infusion one can observe the QT and if it gets too long or arrhythmias develop (proarrhythmia) you can stop the drug. But the half-life is 12 hours, so if a patient gets into trouble (proarrhythmia develops) it takes hours for sotalol to dissipate. Thus, an IV load can reduce hospitalization from three days of observation to one, but it really does not help much when the drug causes life-threatening toxicity. There are "fast on", "fast off" drugs that are modified versions of longer acting drugs. So, a possible solution to the IV Sotalol pro-arrhythmia problem is to modify the sotalol molecule by introducing an ester linkage in a critical part of the molecule. The body has ubiquitous esterase's circulating in the blood stream and they quickly bread down the molecule, reducing the half-life of the drug to minutes. Thus, an ester of sotalol can dissipate rapidly when an infusion is terminated, stopping the QT form further lengthening, no longer perpetuating the arrhythmia the drug has caused. Applying the successful chemical modification of known agents to a clinical problem may offer an innovative solution affording a safer initial loading of sotalol to predict possible long-term toxicity of chronic oral sotalol therapy.

Hospital Re-Admission for Heart Failure

Heart failure is a major clinical problem. In the last two decades the mortality has been greatly reduced with pharmacologic therapy. However, patients with severe heart failure still have a high mortality with multiple hospital admissions. Being hospitalized takes valuable time of the patient away from their activities and their loved ones. Additionally, the cost of hospitalization is very significant. This has led CMS (Center for Medicare and Medicaid Services) to penalize hospitals if the 30-day re-admission for heart failure is greater than the mean admission rate with a 3% reduction in Medicare reimbursements. Thus, hospitals are incentivized not to admit heart failure patients within 30 days of discharge. Lots of research has been undertaken to identify patients that are high risk for early re-admission. Changing in-hospital therapeutics or following outpatients post-discharge for signs of early onset of heart failure have been proposed as possible solutions to the readmission problem. The hope is to treat patients early as outpatients, thus avoiding early re-hospitalization with hospitals being financially penalized. Unfortunately, at best these approaches have resulted in marginal improvement. One factor that greatly effects outcome is patient compliance with effective therapies. Patient non-compliance can be due to the patient's volition or to other factors not under the patient's control. My experience over the years has been that it is difficult for patients to obtain medications in the hospital that are newly prescribed to take home with them. At best patients receive discharge prescriptions to obtain new therapy. Some therapies may need pre-approval by insurance companies and patients may not be up to waiting at an outpatient pharmacy for several hours to have the prescription filled. Some hospitals don't have outpatient pharmacies and patients may not have someone to submit and obtain the newly prescribed medications at a pharmacy immediately after discharge. Family members may bring the prescription to a pharmacy and pick up the prescription days later. One can hypothesize that the re-admission for heart failure is due to a lack of continuity of medications with some being lost or utilization delayed post-discharge. This is a novel hypothesis different from the direction most investigators have been studying. It's a difficult hypothesis to test since records of prescriptions are kept in different places. One would need to obtain hospital medical records of medication and compare these records to outpatient pharmacy records of prescription fills. Adding to the problem is that patients utilize many different outpatient pharmacies to fill the prescriptions they receive. Correlating these records with patient's discharge medications is possible but difficult. Pharmacy records are not easily shared and there is no one database where such information is kept. Testing the hypothesis may be difficult but it does represent a different approach from the prevailing research and if confirmed can lead to improved patient care.

Intellectual Property

When one has an innovative research idea one needs to consider protecting the idea. Some don't want to profit off the innovation and askew pursuing intellectual property protection. Unfortunately, the lack of intellectual property protection can destroy an innovative research idea and its development. Intellectual Property (IP) protection provides exclusivity for the therapy, deice, algorithm, treatment plan or other creation that is new and novel. If IP protection is obtained, then perhaps it may turn out to be economically valuable with the potential for profit. Without the promise of economic viability and profit, drugs or therapeutic approaches can't find funding for development. Even if the NIH supports the research, how will the idea be commercialized and marketed. If a competitor can enter the market, copying the idea while spending a fraction of the capital that was required to develop the product initially investors will refuse to support such a project. Lack of intellectual property severely diminishes the interest in investing in a new idea. Thus, all researchers should give thought to IP protection. Most institutions have an office dealing with intellectual property to assist the investigator as well as the institution. One must be cautious in that Intellectual Property officers are primarily looking out for the institution's interest, not the idea or the innovator, though often all interests may coincide. Individual investigators can protect their work initially using a Provisional Patent which gives priority for the invention to the individual or individuals that receives the provisional patent. This instrument is easily filed and at minimal cost. It gives a year of protection. If the idea is worth pursuing further, then a patent can be filed. This unfortunately becomes more expensive and complicated and in time will require a “national phase” if appropriate with patents filed in various countries, a costly proposition. Still, initially protecting one’s idea is advisable through a Provisional Patent hoping to gain time to obtain financing and support for a patent application and further development.

Summary

As we see from the preceding chapters, an idea needs to be formulated into a hypothesis and then tested using the tools of clinical research. It is a long and difficult process, but one that can be most rewarding and worth undertaking.

Index

C

D

E

F

G

H

I

J

K

L

M

P

Q

R

S

T

U

V

W

X

Y

Z

Made in United States
Orlando, FL
05 November 2026

90229828R10171